DOCUMENTATION FOR PHYSICAL THERAPIST ASSISTANTS

DOCUMENTATION FOR PHYSICAL THERAPIST ASSISTANTS

Marianne Lukan, MA, BS, PT
Instructor
Physical Therapist Assistant Program
Lake Superior College
Duluth, Minnesota

F. A. DAVIS COMPANY·PHILADELPHIA

F.A. Davis Company
1915 Arch Street
Philadelphia, PA 19103

Printed in the United States of America

Last digit indicates print number: 10 9 8 7 6 5 4

Publisher, Allied Health: Jean-François Vilain
Developmental Editor: Crystal Spraggins
Production Editor: Glenn L. Fechner
Cover Designer: Steven R. Morrone

As new scientific information becomes available through basic and clinical research, recommended treatments and drug therapies undergo changes. The author and publisher have done everything possible to make this book accurate, up to date, and in accord with accepted standards at the time of publication. The author, editors, and publisher are not responsible for errors or omissions or for consequences from application of the book, and make no warranty, expressed or implied, in regard to the contents of the book. Any practice described in this book should be applied by the reader in accordance with professional standards of care used in regard to the unique circumstances that may apply in each situation. The reader is advised always to check product information (package inserts) for changes and new information regarding dose and contraindications before administering any drug. Caution is especially urged when using new or infrequently ordered drugs.

Library of Congress Cataloging-in-Publication Data

Lukan, Marianne, 1940-
    Documentation for physical therapist assistants / Marianne Lukan.
        p.   cm.
    Includes bibliographical references and index.
    ISBN 0-8036-0187-5
    1. Physical therapist assistants.   2. Physical therapy—Documentation.   3. Medical records.   I. Title.
    [DNLM: 1. Physical Therapy.   2. Forms and Records Control—standards.   3. Medical Records—standards.
4. Allied Health
Personnel—education.   WB 460 L953d 1997]
RM713.L85   1997
615.8′2—dc20
DNLM/DLC
for Library of Congress   96-20735

To my husband, John, for unending patience and support and for relinquishing hours of relaxation time on the computer.

Preface

The role of the PT is evolving into evaluator, consultant, and manager, with less emphasis and time on daily patient treatment. The PT is ultimately responsible for the patient's treatment program and progress, but the actual provision of treatment and the supervision of the patient's progress can be placed in the hands of the PTA. The PT is accountable to the patient and family, the physician, and the insurance company paying for the physical therapy services. The PTA is directly accountable to the PT. Clear and relevant progress notes must be written by the PTA for good communication between the PT and the PTA, and ultimately among all caregivers involved with the patient's medical care. Insurance reimbursement depends not only on the PT's evaluations and treatment plans, but also on the progress notes written by the PTA. The PTA must have the skills to provide quality physical therapy care and to produce quality documentation.

Documentation for Physical Therapist Assistants was written for the PTA student. This text focuses on the theories and skills the PTA needs to write quality progress notes. It is written with the assumption that the student has minimal knowledge of the medical field, physical therapy treatment procedures, or clinical conditions and that the student is in the beginning courses of the PTA program.

The documentation texts that are presently available provide much of the same information the reader will find in this text, but those texts are directed to the physical therapist. They apply documentation theories and criteria to the problem-solving approach for performing and writing physical therapy evaluations. This text applies documentation theories and criteria to writing progress notes and relating the progress note information to the evaluation performed by the physical therapist. The role of the PTA as a member of the PT/PTA team is woven throughout the content. This text is relevant to the student PTA and the PTA educator, and it could be used as a resource for the PT educator for teaching about the PT/PTA team.

The content of this text is based on three themes:
1. **Documentation is a record of quality of care.** The text uses the *Guidelines for Physical Therapy Documentation,* published by the American Physical Therapy Association, as the resource for standards of quality care and documentation (see Appendix F).
2. **The medical record is a legal record.** The student is reminded that the medical record is likely to be read by a lawyer or jury member in the event of a lawsuit. References regarding legal documentation are used.
3. **Reimbursement is based on the documentation.** Ideally the student should not be taught that this is the *primary* reason for producing quality documentation. *The primary purpose of documentation is to record the evidence of the quality of the care that was provided.* Reality, however, tells us that physical therapy financial survival depends on our documentation. Understanding this should motivate the student to study documentation skills seriously.

Documentation requirements are dynamic, changing as health care insurance changes. Documentation criteria and formats vary from one physical therapy facility to the next. The content in this text is intended to be basic and "generic" so that it can be applied and adapted to documentation formats presently in use and to new formats that may arise in the future. This is not a book on how to write SOAP notes. The intent is to instruct the PTA student in the presentation of the progress note information so that it is organized logically, relevant to the treatment session(s), and supportive of the effectiveness of the treatment plan and goals or outcomes in the initial PT evaluation. Because the SOAP format is presently the most commonly used method for organizing the information, it is referenced frequently in the text, but other models for information organization are included.

The reader will notice that the examples of progress notes throughout this text do not illustrate all of the guidelines for writing the content as discussed in Chapter 4. The use of spaces between the sections of the note and a line separating the problem from the note is a presentation style chosen by the editors of F.A. Davis Company.

To aid learning, the student will find review exercises at the end of each chapter and practice exercises at the end of Chapters 2 through 10. The practice exercises address all the documentation guidelines presented in the text. Chapter 10 can be used as a study guide, as it presents the primary points from each chapter in an outline form. Answers to the review exercises and the practice exercises are in Appendixes D and E. Although the use of abbreviations is discouraged, abbreviations are used in some of the examples and practice exercises. (See Chapter 4 for a discussion on the pitfalls of abbreviation usage.) Abbreviations used in this text are defined in Appendix A. A glossary of terms used in this text is in the back of the book. The student should also consult medical dictionaries and medical terminology resources for definitions of unfamiliar terms.

I have consistently used the term "patient" throughout the text for ease in writing this book. However, many people disapprove of this term because they feel that it implies inappropriate medical passivity and submissiveness. The term "client" is popular now, especially in outpatient clinics, because it suggests that the individual plays an active role as the customer and consumer of our physical therapy services. In long-term care facilities the term "resident" is often used.

As a PTA educator, I have found that the topic of documentation is often viewed as unappealing by many PTA students. This text offers the student an opportunity to learn about the responsibilities of documentation in a relaxed and easy-to-understand manner.

Acknowledgments

Although I worked alone composing and typing the manuscript, this book is the result of support and help from many people. The words "thank you" are not adequate to fully express my gratitude and appreciation for everyone who helped with words of encouragement, with ideas, with contributions, and with criticisms.

A special thanks goes to Marilyn Woods for the hours we spent together going over the wording of the manuscript and for her contributions of case scenarios and forms. I am especially grateful for her experience, insight, and vision regarding documentation and our changing health care system.

"Thank you" to my reviewers, especially Elizabeth F. Burke, MS, PT; Phyllis Beck, PT, MEd; Lynn Lippert MS, PT; William B. Inverso, Jr., PT; Carol A. Maritz, MS, PT; and Stefanie D. Palma, PT, BS, MEd. Their suggestions were insightful and extremely valuable.

"Thank you" to everyone who contributed examples and ideas. I can acknowledge many by name, but I received help from other individuals anonymously. Contributors I can name are Jennifer Warren, Joann Howitz, Deborah L. Miller, Kathleen Johnson, Jeanne Hall, Kathy Kenna, Debi Steinbach, Judith Pautler, Annette Pohl, Kathy Hanson, Susan Sisola, Denise Wise, and Diane Palmstein. I especially appreciate the support, encouragement, and suggestions from the PTA educators who attended the colloquiums in Philadelphia and Minneapolis.

"Thank you" to Jean-François Vilain, publisher, F.A. Davis, and Crystal Spraggins, developmental editor, for their gentle guidance, encouragement, and most important, patience.

A special thanks goes to my son, Jim, for helping me learn WordPerfect for Windows and for the sound bytes and wallpaper programmed into the computer. I loved the surprises and opportunities to laugh during my hours of typing.

ML

Reviewers

Phyllis Beck, PT, MEd
Associate Professor
Physical Therapist Assistant Program
Illinois Central College
East Peoria, Illinois

Elizabeth F. Burke, MS, PT
Professor
Physical Therapist Assistant Program
Springfield Technical Community College
Northampton, Massachusetts

Barbara Gresham, MS, PT
Program Director
Physical Therapist Assistant Program
McLennan Community College
Waco, Texas

William B. Inverso, Jr., PT
Program Director
Physical Therapist Assistant Program
Medical College of Pennsylvania and
   Hahnemann University
Philadelphia, Pennsylvania

Laurie Ihde Larson, BS, PT
Director and Instructor
Physical Therapist Assistant Program
South Central Technical College
Albert Lea Campus
Albert Lea, Minnesota

Lynn Lippert, MS, PT
Director
Physical Therapist Assistant Program
Mount Hood Community College
Gresham, Oregon

Carol A. Maritz, MS, PT
Instructor/Assistant Program Director
Physical Therapist Assistant Program
Medical College of Pennsylvania and
   Hahnemann University
Philadelphia, Pennsylvania

Stephanie D. Palma, PT, BS, MEd
Program Director
Physical Therapist Assistant Program
Department of Physical Therapy
Gwinnet Technical Institute
Lawrenceville, Georgia

Contents

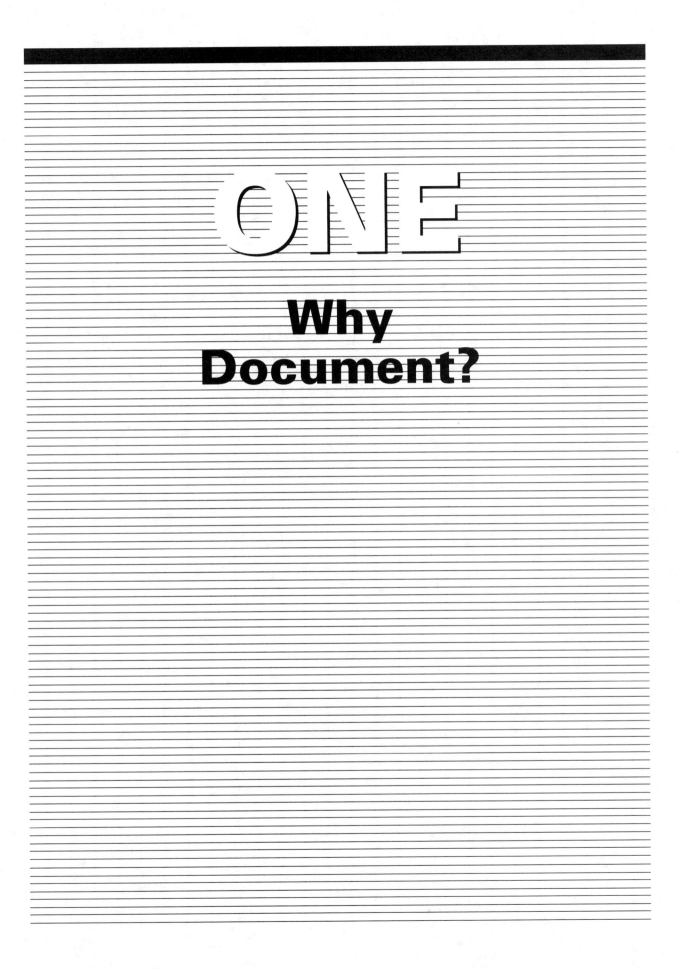

ONE

Why
Document?

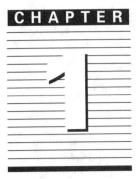
Introduction to Documentation

Learning Objectives
After studying this chapter, the student will be able to:
- Define documentation
- Describe the changes in referral for physical therapy that have occurred during the past 35 years
- Recognize how changes in referral for physical therapy influenced the evolution of the responsibilities of the PT and the PTA
- Recognize the major factor presently influencing the provision of health care services and PT/PTA responsibilities
- Describe the role of documentation in patient care
- Discuss how documentation benefits the PTA, patient, and PT profession

As an educator, I frequently hear students tell me they chose to become PTAs and work with patients daily because they had heard that PTs spend all their time doing evaluations and completing paperwork. However, thorough and proper documentation is the responsibility of *both* the PT and the PTA. This book discusses the documentation tasks that are expected from the PTA, the importance of quality documentation, and the way to produce thorough and proper documentation.

**DEFINITION OF
DOCUMENTATION**

Webster's Dictionary defines document as "anything written that gives information or supplies evidence." Documentation is defined as "the assembling of documents, the using of documentary evidence to support original written work, or the evidence itself . . . , the classifying and making available of knowledge as a procedure." (p. 276).[1]

Evidence of Patient Care

In any health care facility, more than one caregiver provides services to the patient. Records or medical charts are kept to record treatments, services performed, and services to be provided. Medical charts provide information that **authenticates** the care given to the patient and the reasons for providing that care. Documentation is written proof that medical care was given to the patient, and this **evidence** is available for future use. If the treatment provided is not documented in the chart, it is assumed the treatment was not provided. "If it isn't written, it didn't happen" is a good rule to remember.

Accountability for Patient Care

The written record is the mechanism through which the caregiver is held **accountable** for the medical care provided. The record is reviewed by the third-party payer to determine the reimbursement value of the medical services, and the information is studied to measure or determine the efficacy of the treatment procedures. The reader of the medical record will find the rationale that supports the medical necessity of the treatment.

IMPORTANCE OF DOCUMENTATION

The impact of poorly written physical therapy documentation is illustrated in the following story based on a true experience of mine that occurred in 1968. The scenario includes some of the topics and information discussed in this text; however, in some cases the scenario only alludes to this information. A practice exercise after the last chapter challenges the reader to identify these topics.

The Experience

The telephone ring startled the baby and interrupted the relaxed after-dinner mood in the kitchen. My husband and I were chatting about the day, my busy patient schedule at the local hospital, and his insurance sales while our 3-month-old baby napped.

Answering the phone, I immediately heard, "I finally found you! You are to be in court in The City 3 days from now to testify for my client, Tony T. Do you remember him? I will meet with you in my office the night before to go over the medical records and your physical therapy notes."

My stomach did a flip-flop and my heart raced! I certainly did remember Tony. I was his physical therapist 5 years ago when I lived in The City. I did not remember all the details of his treatments, and the thought of testifying at a jury trial stuck terror in my heart! The lawyer assured me that he had my progress notes, and I would have time to review them before I was called to testify.

Settled in the lawyer's office, I looked over Tony's medical chart, which contained a record of his medical care when he was in the hospital and when he came to the physical therapy department as an outpatient. I reviewed the notes I had written about his physical therapy evaluations and treatment (Fig. 1–1). This documentation was in my familiar, illegible handwriting. My notes were only two to three lines in length, and as I read them, they actually told me nothing. There was my signature, or rather not my signature, but just the initials of my name when I was single. I marveled at how the lawyer started with those initials and proceeded to find me, married, and living in another part of the state!

Tony had dived into a shallow pool, hit his head on the bottom, and fractured a vertebra in his neck. This caused some damage to his spinal cord, but it was not completely severed. Tony had quadriparesis, weakness of varying degrees in his arms, legs, and trunk. He gradually improved, and his therapy consisted of exercises and activities to improve the strength, coordination, and endurance needed for him to become independent in all his functional activities. Left with disability, he was suing the owners of the pool. The opposition was fighting to keep the settlement low. They thought there was evidence that he could have been more cooperative and conscientious with his physical therapy.

My documentation followed the format commonly used by therapists in the hospital at that time. These progress notes certainly wouldn't meet Medicare or another third-party payer's criteria now! How was I going to respond to cross-examination by the opposing lawyer, when my notes simply said "pt. improving" and "pt. tolerated treatment well"? They didn't help me recall the specifics of Tony's physical therapy treatments that I needed in order to testify. How I wished these notes had been better written! Somehow, we deciphered the notes, I recalled the information, and I was ready to testify.

My thoughts during my trip home were consumed by the importance of quality docu-

Standardized Record Form Developed By Northeastern Washington Hospital Council

DATE	NOTE: PROGRESS OF CASE, COMPLICATIONS, CONSULTATIONS, CHANGE IN DIAGNOSIS, CONDITION ON DISCHARGE, INSTRUCTIONS TO PATIENT.
8-23-63	Pt is a 6'3 quadraplegic, 17 yr old male. ROM performed. Hamstring tightness. Some tightness in finger extension. Good strength in shoulder girdle muscles, (R) F. tricep, (L) Trace ___ tricep, (R) F. hip flexion. Pt. cooperative. ROM, APT
9-15-63	Pt. states he feels better. Improvement progressing. Pt independently wheeled w/c today. ROM
10-1-63	Pt stood in // bars today, wearing long leg braces. Good (R) tricep, F (L) tricep, finger flex + ext F. ROM, APT
10-26-63	Pt ambulating with Lofstrand crutches and long leg braces. ROM APT
1-3-64	Pt D/C today. Ambulating with short leg brace on (L), Lofstrand crutches. Has home exercise program. To come as OP. ROM APT
2-8-64	Pt continues to improve. ROM RPT

T. T.

PROGRESS NOTES

GOOD BUSINESS FORMS CO SPOKANE   (23504)

FIGURE 1–1 A page from the medical chart containing the physical therapy progress notes for Tony T. written before 1968.

mentation. My court experience would have been so much easier if I had written my notes then in the same format as I do now. What a difference! (Definitions of the abbreviations in the following note are in Appendix A.)

2-8-64:   Pt. has attended outpatient physical therapy 10× since hospital d/c, no-show for appts 1-16, 23, 25, and 2-6-64.

S: Pt. c/o his legs feel "tighter" than usual, states he stopped doing his home exercises because "they're boring, would rather play chess." He doesn't know why he did not come to all his therapy appointments.

O: Pt. ambulates ① using R forearm crutch & L AFO. He demonstrates occasional loss of balance but able to ① regain the balance & does not fall. He circumducts his L leg during initial and mid-swing with inadequate hip and knee flexion. Hypertonus in hip extensor & quadriceps muscles palpable. Active SLR 0–50° bilaterally, 0–30° last week. Pt. uses 5 lb cuff wt. for 30 reps active knee flexion bilaterally, in prone position, up 1 lb from last week. Following 15 sec of pelvic rotation and wt. shifting movements, pt. able to use hip & knee flexion during gait to step over cuff wts lying on the floor. Pt. instructed to always do a few rotational and wt. shifting movements just prior to walking to ↓ mm tone. Pt. ambulated c̄ straight cane, min. assist for balance control, 100 ft on tiled level surface. Pt. correctly demonstrated home ex. program modified to include walking while wearing cuff wts, beginning with 2 lb, & doing concentric and eccentric ex. on stairs. Please refer to written instructions in chart.

MMT finger flexion/extension	2-8-64	1-3-64
right	F	F
left	P	P

Exercises include using his chess set containing the lightest wt. pieces, then progressing to his set with heavier pieces to strengthen finger flexion.

A: Improvement in pt.'s hamstring strength and ability to control extensor hypertonus to improve quality of gait. Potential for meeting goal of Ⓘ community ambulation c̄ straight cane is good. Finger strength status quo, possibly due to not exercising. Exercises changed to be more interesting and motivating for pt.

P: Pt. scheduled 2×/week for 2 weeks to monitor home exercise program & ambulation progress. Will focus on ambulation c̄ cane on stairs, carpet, and grass next session.

—Marianne Mouser, PT Lic. #123

EVOLUTION OF PT/PTA RESPONSIBILITIES AND ROLE OF DOCUMENTATION

The story of the 1968 event gives an example of how documentation has evolved over time. This change has been a result of the changing responsibilities of the PT and the PTA.

The Past

Changes in physician referral for physical therapy and the enactment of Medicare insurance are two events in history that have influenced the evolution of PT and PTA treatment and documentation responsibilities and the role of documentation in patient care.

Changes in Physician Referral for Physical Therapy

The method by which physicians prescribe physical therapy has changed throughout the profession's short history. The changes have increased the PT's clinical decision-making power, led to the development of the physical therapy diagnosis or problem, and offered the opportunity for autonomy.

THE PHYSICAL THERAPY PRESCRIPTION   Until the early 1960s, patients came to a PT with referrals from physicians that were in the form of physical therapy prescriptions. That is, they read much like a medication prescription, as illustrated in Figure 1–2, or the instructions were more general (i.e., ultrasound, massage, exercise). The PT was required to follow the physician's orders and to provide the treatment as prescribed. If the PT did not agree with the treatment plan, he or she needed to discuss this with the physician in an attempt to agree upon a more appropriate treatment plan. The PT was not always successful in convincing the physician to change the order; thus, the physical therapy treatment provided may not have been as effective as possible. The PT's responsibilities were at a technician level, following exact directions from the physician. The PT documented briefly that the treatment was provided and whether or not the patient was improving.

EVALUATE AND TREAT   In the early 1960s, PTs began convincing some physicians that PTs had the training and knowledge to evaluate a patient's neuromusculoskeletal system and to determine the treatment appropriate for the patient's condition. Patients brought referrals from their physicians that provided the diagnosis and stated "evaluate and treat." The responsibil-

> ### P. T. Knowes, MD
> *123 Medical Building*
> *Yourtown, AZ 12345*
> *(001) 222-3333*
>
> Physical Therapy for Hazel Jones
>
> US at 1.5 w/cm² for 5 min to the right deltoid insertion, followed by 10 min of massage.
> AAROM 10 reps for abduction, flexion, and external rotation.
>
> *P.T. Knowes, MD*

FIGURE 1–2 Illustration of a physician's order for physical therapy that tells the PT exactly what to do. It resembles a medication prescription.

ity of the PT expanded to include (1) determining the physical therapy problem based on results of the evaluation findings and (2) defining the treatment plan. The physical therapy problem would be described in terms of the neuromusculoskeletal abnormality, and the treatment plan would be directed toward correcting or minimizing this problem. The PT needed to have evaluation skills to identify physical therapy problems and to make clinical decisions regarding the treatment of those problems. Writing the initial, interim, and discharge evaluations became additional documentation responsibilities.

The first academic program for training the PTA was established in 1967. The PTA became the technician providing the physical therapy treatments under the direct guidance and supervision of the PT. Writing progress notes was a documentation responsibility shared by the PT and PTA.

DIRECT ACCESS   Direct access allows a person access to the medical care system directly through a PT. The PT may evaluate the patient to determine whether the patient's condition is a neuromusculoskeletal disorder treatable by physical therapy without a physician's referral. Nebraska has allowed direct access since 1957, and California eliminated the physician's referral requirement in 1968. When Maryland's Physical Therapy Practice Act was amended in 1979 to allow direct access, many American Physical Therapy Association (APTA) state chapters launched their amendment campaigns. Today, a majority of states have direct access, and the remaining states have direct access legislation in progress.

Direct access gives the PT opportunity for autonomy, but it also requires the PT to have the skills and knowledge to recognize conditions that are *not* indicative of physical therapy problems. It is the responsibility of the PT to refer a patient to a physician or another appropriate health care provider if there are signs and symptoms of a systemic disorder or a problem that is beyond the scope or expertise of the PT. *It is the PTA's responsibility to report to the PT any signs or symptoms or lack of progress that would indicate a need for PT reevaluation or referral.*

PT education has had to change focus to increase the emphasis on scientific knowledge, evaluation skills, and critical thinking and research and to decrease the emphasis on treatment skills. The training of the PTA, while focusing on treatment skills, has expanded to emphasize the theories behind the treatment skills. This provides the PTA with the knowledge to make clinical decisions within the parameters of the PT treatment plan and PTA scope of practice. In some areas, PTA responsibilities have evolved such that PTAs are able to treat patients when the PT is not on the premises but accessible by telephone.

Establishment of Medicare   Before 1970, documentation in the medical chart was not always thorough or specific. Health care providers knew documentation should be done well, but unfortunately poor-quality documentation was not difficult to find. Progress notes were typically brief, one or two lines, and of a subjective and/or judgmental nature. For example: "Patient feeling better today" (see Fig.

1–1). There were no standards for documentation, and those paying the health care bills did not demand accountability for those bills. This changed in the mid-1960s when Health Insurance for the Aged and Disabled Act, known as Medicare, was enacted. The federal government was purchasing medical care for the elderly. Within the Department of Health and Human Services, the Health Care Financing Administration (HCFA) issued standards for documentation to be followed for all patients on Medicare. Other insurance companies followed Medicare's example. Those paying the medical bills demanded that health care providers be *accountable* for the dollars being spent. This accountability was determined through proper documentation that clearly identified the physical therapy problem, the treatment goals, the treatment plans, and the treatment results.

The Present

At the present time, the 1990s, our health care system is in a state of transition as the provision of services is modified to function with limited financial resources. The physical therapy provider is placed in a position of competing for these limited funds. Physical therapy services will not be financed if the treatments are not effective and efficient. The patient or client seeks physical therapy because a neuromusculoskeletal problem prevents the individual from **functioning** in his or her environment. The treatment goal is directed toward improving or restoring the patient's functional abilities by minimizing or resolving the neuromusculoskeletal problem. This needs to be accomplished in a cost-effective manner. Documentation that meets today's standards provides the basis for research to measure functional outcomes and to identify the most effective and efficient treatment procedures. Documentation now must describe what functional activities the individual has difficulty performing and show how the treatment procedures are effective in improving or restoring the patient's function. Documentation *must* be done properly if the physical therapy health care provider is to survive financially.

ROLE OF DOCUMENTATION IN PATIENT CARE

Three themes are repeated in this text: (1) documentation records the **quality** of patient care; (2) documentation constructs a **legal report** of patient care; and (3) documentation provides the basis for **reimbursement** for the patient care.

A Record of the Quality of Patient Care

The term **quality care** is used in this text to mean medical care that is appropriate for and focused on the patient's problems relevant to the diagnosis or reason the individual is receiving the care. Quality physical therapy care is defined as care that follows the *Standards of Practice* criteria for physical therapy published by APTA.[2]

To provide quality medical care, there must be good **communication** among caregivers. The PTA *must* communicate with the PT. The PTA may also share and coordinate information with other providers of the medical services the patient is receiving: other PTs and PTAs who may fill in when the PTA is absent—occupational therapists and occupational therapy assistants, nurses and nursing assistants, physicians and physician assistants, speech pathologists, psychologists, social workers, and chaplains—to name a few. The medical record is the avenue through which the medical team communicates regarding (1) identification of the patient's problems, (2) solutions, (3) plans for the patient's discharge, and (4) coordination of the continuum of care. This communication process helps to ensure quality of care.

Ensuring Quality of Care

A record review process and use of the findings serve as methods for monitoring and influencing the quality of care provided by the medical facility. The information in the medical record is audited or reviewed for three purposes: (1) quality assurance, (2) research and education, and (3) reimbursement.

1. Records are reviewed to determine whether the health care provided meets **standards and criteria.** This is done *externally* by agencies accrediting the facility and *internally* by a quality assurance committee. Problem areas are identified, and plans are made for correction and improvement. This is a continuous process; the committee usually meets monthly, and facilities are accredited every 5 to 10 years. PTAs are permitted to serve on the quality assurance committee.
2. The information in the medical record is used for **research** and student **learning.** Research helps to validate treatment techniques and to identify new and better ways to provide health care. The record is used for retrospective studies that measure outcomes

to determine the most cost-effective treatment approach to patient care. Students are encouraged to question and challenge treatment procedures as part of their learning process.

3. The third-party payers such as insurance companies and Medicare decide how to reimburse for the medical care provided by reading the documentation in the medical record. *The record must show that the patient's problems were identified and treatment was directed toward goals of solving those problems and discharging the patient.*

Documentation Standards and Criteria

Documentation should follow standards and criteria set by a variety of sources. The standards are similar, but the PTA should be familiar with the criteria required by (1) the federal government, (2) the state government, (3) professional agencies, (4) accrediting agencies, and (5) the health care facility.

THE FEDERAL GOVERNMENT   The federal government funds and administers Medicare. The PTA must follow Medicare documentation requirements when treating a patient who has this insurance. These requirements change frequently and can become complicated. The PTA must stay informed and up-to-date in his or her knowledge of Medicare requirements.

THE STATE GOVERNMENT   Although funded by the federal government, Medicaid is administered by the state. The state government funds medical assistance and worker's compensation and will have documentation requirements for patients who have these insurances. The state may ask that specific data from the medical record be reported annually. Other documentation criteria determined at the state level may be influenced by the state's physical therapy legislation. The PTA must be well informed about his or her state's Physical Therapy Practice Act.

PROFESSIONAL AGENCIES   Professional agencies recommend documentation standards, such as the APTA's *Guidelines for Physical Therapy Documentation*.[3] These standards are the basis for the documentation instructions in this text and can be found in Appendix F.

ACCREDITING AGENCIES   Accrediting agencies provide standards that health care facilities must follow to meet accreditation criteria. Hospitals are accredited by the Joint Commission on Accreditation of Healthcare Organizations (JCAHO), and rehabilitation facilities are accredited by the Commission on Accreditation of Rehabilitation Facilities (CARF).

THE HEALTH CARE FACILITY   Each health care facility has individual documentation criteria and will incorporate federal, state, and professional standards into its own procedures. The PTA can follow all standards and criteria by remembering this good rule: *Follow the policies and procedures at the facility where you work.*

A Legal Record

The medical record is a legal document and legal proof of the quality of care provided. The record *protects* the patient and the caregivers should any question arise in the future regarding the patient's care. Health care providers work under the shadow of a possible malpractice lawsuit. Patients do become dissatisfied, and questions about the care provided may arise months or years after the patient received treatment. Many patients' cases go to court because their injury or illness was caused by an accident or negligence on the part of someone else. PTs are often called to testify in court. It is possible even for the PTA to be called. Providing safe and thorough patient care is the *best* protection against being sued for malpractice. Clear and accurate documentation is the best defense if the PT or PTA is called to testify.

A Basis for Reimbursement

The insurance company or organization paying for medical services determines the reimbursement rate from the information recorded in the medical chart. Payment is often denied when the documentation does not clearly provide the rationale to support the medical care that was provided. Under some insurance plans, the caregiver must provide effective patient care while containing the costs within a preset payment amount. The caregiver demonstrates accountability for these costs by thorough and proper documentation of the care provided.

SUMMARY   Documenting in the medical record is one of the many duties of the PTA. The medical record is a legal document that proves that medical care was given and holds the health care providers accountable for the quality of the care given. It is an avenue for constant communication among caregivers so that goals can be identified and the treatment progress monitored. Insurance representatives read the medical record to determine whether or not to reimburse for the medical services provided.

Historically, PTs were technicians, providing physical therapy treatments that were prescribed in detail by the physician. Responsibilities have evolved such that PTs are now evaluators, consultants, managers, and practitioners seeing patients (clients) without a physician's referral. PTAs provide treatment under the guidance and supervision of the PT.

Financial resources to fund health care are no longer readily available. Physical therapy services must be provided in an efficient and cost-effective manner. The treatment goal now must focus on improving the client's functional abilities. Research must be done to measure outcomes or results of physical therapy procedures to define the most effective and efficient treatments that will accomplish the functional goals. Proper documentation will facilitate this research.

The provision of up-to-date and valid physical therapy services will be ensured through documentation that follows standards and criteria determined by federal and state governments, professional agencies, accrediting agencies, and the individual clinical facility. Documenting according to standards and legal guidelines will produce a medical record that protects the patient and the PTA if the medical record is used in court proceedings. Documentation formats differ from facility to facility, but all incorporate the professional standards and criteria. The PTA should follow the policies and procedures of his or her clinical facility.

REFERENCES
1. Cayne, BS (ed): The New Lexicon Webster's Dictionary of the English Language. Lexicon Publications, New York, 1989, p 276.
2. American Physical Therapy Association: Standards of Practice. APTA, Alexandria, VA, June 1992.
3. American Physical Therapy Association: Guidelines for Physical Therapy Documentation. APTA, Alexandria, VA, March 1993.

REVIEW EXERCISES

1. Describe what is meant by the following rule: "If it isn't written, it didn't happen."

2. Describe the changes in referral for physical therapy that have occurred during the past 35 years.

3. Discuss how changes in referral for physical therapy influenced the evolution of the responsibilities of the PT and the PTA.

4. Define direct access.

5. Identify the major factor presently influencing the provision of health care services and PT/PTA responsibilities.

6. Describe three purposes for the medical record.

7. Explain why the medical record is audited.

8. Identify who determines standards or criteria for documentation.

9. Explain why the PTA should use the rule "follow the policies and procedures at the facility where you work."

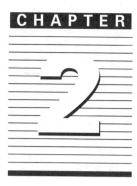

CHAPTER

2

Documentation Content

Learning Objectives
After studying this chapter, the student will be able to:
- Identify the six categories of documentation content
- Briefly describe the content in each category
- Differentiate PT and PTA documentation responsibilities
- Discuss physical therapy evaluations, the types, and PTA involvement

The medical record is the written account of the patient's medical care. The content describes the medical care provided from the moment the patient is admitted to the medical facility to the moment he or she is discharged from the facility.

**CONTENT
CATEGORIES**

Documentation content can be grouped into six categories:
1. **Data** relevant to the patient's condition
2. The **problem(s)** requiring medical treatment
3. **Treatment plan or action** to address the problem(s)

4. **Goals or outcomes** of the treatment plan
5. **Record of administration of the treatment plan**
6. **Treatment effectiveness** or results of the treatment plan

This information is found in the written evaluations, in the progress notes, and in the recording of specialized test results such as x-ray and laboratory reports. A brief description of each content area is presented in this chapter to provide an overview of the content of the medical record. In-depth explorations of these content areas for physical therapy documentation are the topics discussed in Chapters 5, 6, 7, and 8.

DATA The information gathered about the patient forms the basis for both subjective and objective data. Most of this information is gathered at the time of admission or the first time the patient is seen by each medical service provider. However, information is always being gathered throughout the time the patient is receiving medical care. Data gathered when the patient is admitted will be located in the initial evaluations performed by the various medical services. For example, a young male student is admitted to the emergency room (ER) at XXX hospital, 2:45 AM Saturday, after being involved in a motorcycle accident. Information is gathered at admission to the ER, when the patient is taken to x-ray, when the patient is admitted to the orthopedic hospital floor, and when laboratory tests are performed. More information will be gathered when the patient is first seen by physical therapy, occupational therapy, and social services. Examples of the data each discipline may want to gather about this patient can be found in Table 2–1.

TABLE 2–1. Examples of Data Gathered by Various Medical Services Treating a Student Involved in a Motorcycle Accident

ADMITTING CLERK

Past admissions to the hospital
Insurance information
Nearest relatives
General information about the accident

PHYSICIAN

Past medical history
More detailed information about the accident
Physical examination results from primary physician
Orthopedic examination results from orthopedic surgeon
Diagnostic test results
Laboratory test results
X-ray results

NURSE

Vital signs
Bowel and bladder function
Skin condition
General nutritional status
General ability to care for self, communicate, and make judgments

PHYSICAL THERAPIST

Flexibility or joint range of motion
Muscle strength
Sensation
Posture
Ability to move about in his environment

OCCUPATIONAL THERAPIST

More specific ability to care for self in activities of daily living
Vocational abilities
Homemaking abilities
General vision, hearing, and communication abilities

SOCIAL WORKER

Home environment and lifestyle
More specific financial concerns
General emotional adjustment
Family support and family adjustment

Subjective Data
Information *told* to the health care provider is subjective data. Some information relevant to the patient's condition and reason for admission to the medical facility is collected by interviewing the patient or significant others. Subjective data include (1) information about the patient's past medical history, (2) the **symptoms** or complaints that caused the patient to seek medical attention, (3) the factors that produced the symptoms, (4) the patient's functional and lifestyle needs, and (5) the patient's goals or expectations from the medical care. Collecting subjective data is an ongoing process while the medical care is being provided. The information reflects both the patient's response to the treatment and the effectiveness of the treatment. The PT and PTA seek information provided by the client. The PT documents subjective data in the physical therapy evaluation reports, and the PTA documents subjective data in the daily or weekly progress notes.

Objective Data
Objective information includes information that is reproducible. Objective information relating to the patient's condition is gathered by careful examination of the patient via assessment methods (e.g., measurements, tests, observations) that can be **reproduced** by any medical professional with the same training as the one performing the examination. Objective data are the **signs** of the patient's condition. Reviewing the signs by repetition of the measurements, tests, and observations is also an ongoing process for determining the treatment effectiveness and patient progress. The PT performs the physical therapy examination or evaluation and uses objective methods to gather data. These data are used to determine the physical therapy diagnosis or problem. The PTA repeats any measurements, tests, and observations within the scope of his or her PTA training to determine the patient's progress toward accomplishing the treatment goals.

THE PROBLEM REQUIRING MEDICAL TREATMENT
The medical team identifies the patient's medical problems based on the data collected in the various evaluations performed by the disciplines. The physician determines the **medical diagnosis,** and other professionals identify the problems that are treatable by their respective disciplines. The diagnosis is documented by the physician in the medical chart, usually near the beginning of the chart in a section specified for the physician's report. The identification of the **physical therapy problem** is usually documented in the physical therapy initial evaluation, located in either the physical therapy section or the evaluation section of the chart. Other problems are discussed in other health care providers' evaluations. Problems that may have been identified by the physicians, nurses, and social worker examining the student in the motorcycle accident include the following:

1. Compound fracture of the shaft of right femur
2. Lacerations into quadriceps muscles
3. Infected open wound
4. Edema of the right foot
5. Questionable chemical dependency
6. Fever
7. Elevated blood pressure

Definition of Terms
It will be helpful to define some terms before comparing the medical diagnoses with the physical therapy problem. Guccione[1] recommends that PTs define the disabling process using the Nagi model. This model describes a chain of events beginning with a **pathology,** which causes or leads to impairments, which cause or lead to functional limitations, which cause or lead to a disability. **Impairments** are defined as "the abnormalities of anatomic, physiologic, or psychologic origin within specific organs or systems of the body."[2] **Functional limitations** are "restrictions or inability to perform activities of daily living (ADL) skills such as transfers, gait, and bed mobility."[2] **Disability** refers to "restriction of or inability to perform a normal range of ADL . . . such as inability to walk, and higher level activities, such as inability to participate in athletic games." (p 83).[2]

The Nagi model is a variation of the model describing the implication of pathology issued by the World Health Organization (WHO). The terminology in this model, the International Classification of Impairments, Disabilities, and Handicaps (ICIDH), is used in the international physical therapy community. The ICIDH term "disability" is equivalent to Nagi's "functional limitation," and the ICIDH term "handicap" has the same meaning as Nagi's "disability."

The Medical Diagnosis

The medical diagnosis is of a systemic disease or disorder, which is determined by the physician's evaluation and diagnostic tests. "Diagnosis is the recognition of disease. It is the determination of the cause and nature of pathologic conditions." (p 2).[3] The medical diagnosis is equivalent to the pathology in the Nagi and ICIDH models. The student in the motorcycle accident was diagnosed as having "a fractured femur and infected lacerations."

The Physical Therapy Problem

The physical therapy problem is *not* a medical diagnosis. According to Sahrmann,[4] the physical therapy problem is the identification of pathokinesiologic (i.e., study of movements related to a given disorder) problems associated with faulty biomechanical or neuromuscular action.[3] The physical therapy problem is the determination of the location and severity of a neuromusculoskeletal abnormality that interferes with a person's ability to perform *functional* tasks. Some call this the physical therapy "diagnosis." This text will refer to the physical therapy **problem** to avoid confusion and to emphasize that the physical therapist does *not* determine the medical diagnoses. The physical therapy problem has two parts: (1) a neuromusculoskeletal dysfunction and (2) a functional limitation. The neuromusculoskeletal dysfunction is the impairment(s). In the Nagi model, the problem consists of the patient's impairments and functional limitations, whereas in the ICIDH model, the problem consists of the patient's impairments and disabilities. In both models, the physical therapy treatment objectives are aimed at eliminating or minimizing the impairments and functional limitations or disabilities. The desired outcome of the physical therapy treatment is preventing or minimizing the severity of the disability or handicap.

Neuromusculo–skeletal Dysfunction

Neuromusculoskeletal dysfunctions are impairments of the bones, joints, ligaments, muscles, and tendons, or problems with movement resulting from a pathology in the brain or spinal cord. A few examples of dysfunctions treatable by a PT include muscle weakness; tendon inflammation; connective tissue tightness, with limited range of motion (ROM) in the joints; muscle spasms; edema; and difficulties moving in bed, moving from sitting to standing, and walking. The neuromusculoskeletal dysfunction in the physical therapy problem may be the same as the medical diagnosis (e.g., "a rotated L5 vertebra," with muscle spasms and pain limiting a truck driver's sitting tolerance to 5 minutes). The physician may determine that the L5 vertebra is rotated on the basis of x-rays and examination and may indicate this as the medical diagnosis. The client or patient may have gone to see the PT first, the PT having performed the evaluation and identified the rotated vertebra. This, plus the muscle spasms, is the neuromusculoskeletal dysfunction part of the physical therapy problem. A patient may have a medical diagnosis *with* a physical therapy problem (e.g., *rheumatoid arthritis with adhesive capsulitis of the anterior capsule limiting shoulder ROM* interfering with a retiree's ability to put on shirt and sweater). In the latter case, rheumatoid arthritis is the medical diagnosis, and *adhesive capsulitis limiting shoulder ROM* is part of the physical therapy problem.

Functional Limitations

The definition of the physical therapy problem must include the patient's **functional abilities or inabilities.** The patient comes to physical therapy because of an inability to function adequately in his or her environment. In the previous examples, the student with the fractured femur will *not be able to ambulate bearing weight on the fractured leg,* the truck driver with the rotated L5 vertebra *cannot sit longer than 5 minutes,* and the retiree with rheumatoid arthritis *cannot put on his shirt and sweater.* These functional problems become the basis for determining the goals toward which the physical therapy treatments are directed, and the rate of progress toward accomplishing the goals determines the duration of the physical therapy services.

Examples

The PTA should distinguish between the **medical diagnosis** and the **physical therapy problem** when treating and documenting. Examples of medical diagnoses include the following:

1. Multiple sclerosis
2. Rheumatoid arthritis
3. Fractured right femur
4. Cerebral vascular accident (CVA) secondary to thrombosis
5. Compression fracture of T12 vertebra with compression of spinal cord

Physical therapy problems that may be associated with the medical diagnoses listed are discussed in the following examples.

Problem: Ataxia of lower extremities with inability to ambulate independently.
Discussion: A patient with the medical diagnosis of multiple sclerosis may have the neuromuscular physical therapy problem of ataxia (the impairment) and the functional problem of inability to ambulate (the functional limitation). In the past, the result of the treatment was documented by a description of the improvement in impairment (e.g., pt.'s coordination improved as pt. able to place R heel on L knee). Today, treatment effectiveness is documented by a description of a decrease in the functional limitation, such as improvement in the ability or quality of the patient's ambulation (e.g., pt. able to walk to mailbox without assistive device but needs standby assist [SBA] because of occasional loss of balance).

Problem: Limited ROM in right shoulder limiting the ability to put on shirt and sweater.
Discussion: The patient with the medical diagnosis of rheumatoid arthritis may have the physical therapy problem consisting of the impairment, limited ROM, and the functional limitation (Nagi) or disability (ICIDH) of difficulty in dressing. In the past, it was acceptable to document treatment effectiveness in degrees of increased ROM (e.g., shoulder flexion 0–100°, an improvement of 20° since initial eval.). Today, a description of the patient's ability to put on his or her shirt or sweater documents the treatment effectiveness (e.g., client able to put on loose-fitting pullover sweater without assistance).

TREATMENT PLAN OR ACTION

The problem list is used to plan the patient's medical treatment. Appropriate strategies for resolving or minimizing the problems are outlined by the various disciplines involved. These strategies are the treatment plans. In the case of the motorcycle accident patient, the physician would design a treatment plan for medication to stop the infection, and then for surgery to pin and stabilize the fractured femur. Nursing may design a treatment plan for positioning the right foot to reduce the edema and for monitoring blood pressure. The social worker may design a treatment plan to help the patient decrease his dependency on alcohol. Later, the PT may design a treatment plan to teach the patient to walk with crutches. In the truck driver example, the PT may design a treatment plan to apply a modality that will relax muscle spasms, to perform mobilization techniques to derotate the L5 vertebra, and to educate the driver about sitting support and posture. These treatment plans are described in the medical record and include frequency and duration of the treatment procedures.

Informed Consent to the Treatment Plan

The treatment plans and purposes for the treatment are explained to the patient and significant others. In some cases, the patient may participate in the designing of the plan. The treatment procedures are described to the patient, and the purposes and expected results of the treatment are explained. The patient is informed of any risks or side effects from the treatment. The patient or a representative for the patient should agree to the treatment plan and procedures. His or her decision to consent to the treatment (**informed consent**) is based on the information provided about the treatment. In many medical facilities, a formal informed consent form or document must be signed before treatment is initiated. When a patient is receiving physical therapy, the PT designs the treatment plan and reviews the plan with the patient. Thus, the appropriate person to obtain the informed consent signature is the PT, *not* the PTA. This signed document is placed in the medical record.

GOALS OR OUTCOMES

All health care providers identify the goals or outcomes to be accomplished by their treatment plans. In the case of the student in the motorcycle accident, the physician's goals may be to treat the infection and to stabilize the fractured femur so that healing can occur. The nurse's goals may be to monitor the patient and to prevent any other problems that may occur as a result of the patient's injury and temporary inactivity. The social worker's goal may be to help the patient find the most appropriate resources and help for his chemical dependency.

The functional goals or outcomes toward which the PT's treatment plan is directed should include the patient's goals (i.e., what is meaningful to the patient). Therefore, the physical therapy goals are planned with patient and PT collaboration. The truck driver's functional outcome is to be able to sit for at least 2 hours so that he can return to work. The student's functional outcome is to learn how to use crutches so that he can return to college. These goals give the PTA direction for planning the treatment sessions, progressing the treatment outlined in the PT's plan, and recommending the termination of the treatment. It is important for the PT and the PTA to stay focused on the purpose of the treatment plan and to aim everything done during a treatment session toward improving or resolving the functional problem that brought the client to physical therapy. Likewise, all documentation should be focused on the treatment appropriate for the goals and on the progress toward accomplishing the functional outcomes.

RECORD OF ADMINISTRATION OF THE TREATMENT PLAN

The medical chart contains proof that the treatment plan is being carried out. Recording the administration of the treatment can range from simply checking off in a flow chart or checklist, to writing a narration or report about the treatment in daily, weekly, or monthly progress notes.

The Progress Note

The progress note is a recording of the treatment provided for each problem, the patient's reaction to treatment, progress toward the goals or outcomes, and any changes in the patient's condition. Although both the PT and the PTA write the progress notes, this text is directed toward the PTA and the skills needed to write quality notes.

TREATMENT EFFECTIVENESS

This content area contains an interpretation of the patient's **response** to the treatments. The caregiver documents whether or not the goals were met, thus documenting the effectiveness of the treatment plan. *This is the most important content in the medical record.* It is the "bottom line" of the health care business. This information tells the reader the quality of the medical care provided. The researcher uses this content to measure outcomes and to determine the efficacy of treatment procedures. The third-party payer reads this information first to determine whether the medical care met the requirements for reimbursement.

DOCUMENTATION RESPONSIBILITIES

The documentation content is found in the evaluations and progress notes. The PT is responsible for the evaluations, consultations, and decision making required for the patient's physical therapy health care. Therefore, the physical therapist's documentation responsibilities are to record the (1) initial evaluation, which includes goals or outcomes and treatment plan; (2) interim or progress evaluations performed; (3) discharge information; and (4) changes in the treatment plan. The PT may also write progress notes. The primary documentation responsibility of the PTA is to record the progress or interim notes.

THE EVALUATION

Before evaluations are discussed, the reader must understand the distinction between **assessment** and **evaluation.** The PTA is trained to assess the patient, not to evaluate the patient. According to the APTA task force on standards in measurement in physical therapy, assessment is defined as "measurement, quantification, or placing a value or label on something. Assessment is often confused with evaluation; an assessment results from the act of assessing." Evaluation is defined as "a judgment based on a measurement; often confused with assessment and examination. Evaluations are judgments of the value or worth of something." (p 595).[5]

PTA Involvement

Although the PTA *does not perform* evaluations, he or she can *assist* the PT with the evaluation procedures. The PTA can take notes and help gather the subjective data. The PTA can take measurements, perform some tests, and record the results, but the PTA may not *interpret* the results. Performing the tests and recording the results constitute the assessment. Interpreting the results involves making a judgment and placing a worth on the results; this is *evaluating.* Examples of tests and measurements that are within the scope of PTA practice are girth measurements, manual muscle testing of muscle groups, goniometry measurements, and vital signs. During the course of a patient's treatment, the PTA often is expected to repeat the measurements and tests to assess the patient's progress since the initial evaluation. These objective data are more reliable when the same person performs the tests and measurements in a consistent manner throughout the course of the patient's treatment. Assisting the PT with the evaluation offers the opportunity for the PTA and patient to become acquainted so that the patient will feel comfortable working with the PTA as the treatment plan is carried out.

The PTA must be familiar with the content of the PT evaluations. The evaluation report informs the PTA of the patient's medical diagnosis and the physical therapy problem. The PTA follows the treatment plan outlined in the evaluation and directs all treatment sessions toward accomplishing the goals or outcomes listed in the evaluation.

Types of Evaluations and the Content

The PT should always perform an **initial evaluation** and a **discharge evaluation** of the patient and may perform one or more **interim evaluations,** depending on the length of time the patient is receiving the physical therapy care. The APTA *Guidelines for Physical Therapy Documentation*[6] outlines the recommended content of the evaluations. A description of each evaluation type follows with a listing of the recommended information contained in the evaluation. The documentation content categories, discussed in this chapter, are indicated in bold next to the evaluation information that is appropriate for each category to demonstrate how the physical therapy evaluation conforms to the documentation content in the medical record.

Initial Evaluation

This evaluation is performed the first time the PT sees the patient. The written report of the initial evaluation contains the following:

1. **Data:** General statistics about the patient given before the evaluation is performed, although this information may be elsewhere in the chart, such as in notes from admissions or the physician.

   Examples: Age, medical diagnosis, name, sex, date of birth (DOB), physician, complications, precautions. All of these data are required in the medical record but may not all be in the PT's evaluation if already located elsewhere in the chart.

2. **Subjective data:** Information the patient tells the PT or PTA during the interview.

   Examples: Onset of injury/disease/pain, chief complaint, location of complaints, functional limitations, home situation, lifestyle, goals, pertinent medical history.

3. **Objective Data:** Results of objective testing and observations.

   Physical Status: Strength, endurance, skin condition, ROM, neurologic status.
   Functional Status: Mobility, transfers, ambulation, ADLs, work/school/home.
   Mental Status: Cognition, orientation; communication problems; judgment; ability to follow directions.

4. PT's interpretation of the testing with identification of the **problem(s).**
5. Short-term and long-term **goals or outcomes** related to resolving the problem(s) written in *functional* terms.
6. **Treatment plans** related to accomplishing the goals and including specific treatment(s), their frequency, and duration.
7. Statement regarding the patient's rehabilitation potential or expectations of treatment effectiveness. An estimate of the length of time the patient will be receiving physical therapy treatment.
8. A schedule or plan for evaluating the effectiveness of the treatment.

Interim or Progress Evaluations

Interim evaluations are performed by the PT periodically throughout the period of time the patient is receiving physical therapy. These should not be confused with the interim or progress *notes* that are written by the PTA. The progress evaluation content includes the following:

1. **Treatment procedures administered:** Summary of past treatment provided

2. **Subjective data:** Patient's subjective information as to the effectiveness of the treatment

3. **Objective data:** A repeat of the testing and observations made in the initial evaluation

4. **Results or effectiveness of treatment plan:**
   a. Interpretation of objective testing and observations and a comparison with the initial evaluation

    b. Statement addressing the accomplishment of goals set in the initial evaluation and any new **goals** set

    c. Information regarding any change in the patient's status

5. **Treatment plan written by the PT:** This indicates whether the initial plan is to be continued or changed

Discharge Evaluation

This is the patient's final evaluation and the final note about the patient in the medical record. *This note must be written by the PT.* The content includes the following:

1. Brief summary of the treatment that was provided (treatment procedures administered)
2. Relevant information provided by the patient (subjective data)
3. Interpretation of repeated testing and observations and a comparison with latest interim evaluation (objective data and results or effectiveness of treatment)
4. Statement regarding accomplishment of short-term goals (STGs) and long-term goals (LTGs) (results or effectiveness of treatment)
5. Further treatment or care needed after discharge
6. Plans for follow-up or monitoring after discharge

Comments About Discharge Notes

There is disagreement among physical therapy professionals about the definition of a discharge evaluation and a discharge summary. Some believe the evaluation and the summary are the same, whereas others consider them different types of documents.

If a discharge summary is considered the same as a discharge evaluation, then the evaluation/summary will have content that interprets the testing results and identifies plans for the patient after discharge. Decisions about the patient's care after discharge may be made based on the information in the discharge evaluation/summary. In this case, only a PT can write a discharge summary.

Some physical therapy clinicians write discharge summaries that only summarize the care given the patient, summarize the patient's response to treatment, and state objectively the functional status of the patient at the time of discharge. No interpretation of the data is made, no plan for the patient's care after discharge is identified, and no decisions are made based on the information. This type of a discharge note can be written by a PTA. If the physical therapy clinician writes discharge summaries of this nature, there still must be a discharge evaluation written by the PT as the *final* note in the patient's medical record.

PTA Use of the Evaluation Content When Documenting

When writing progress notes, the PTA refers to the problems, goals, and treatment plans in the initial and interim evaluations. Progress notes should record the effectiveness of treatment by comparing the patient's progress toward accomplishing the goals with the status of the patient at initial evaluation.

SUMMARY

The information documented in the medical record consists of (1) data relevant to the patient's condition, (2) problems that require medical attention, (3) a treatment plan to address the problems, (4) goals of the treatment plan, (5) a record of the administration of the treatments, and (6) results or effectiveness of the treatment plan.

A comparison of the medical diagnosis with the physical therapy problem was presented. The physical therapy problem is the identification of the location and severity of a biomechanical or neuromusculoskeletal abnormality causing a functional limitation. The functional limitation is the primary reason the patient seeks physical therapy, and improvement of this limitation is the goal of the physical therapy treatment.

Information about the treatment procedures, its purposes, expected results, and any possible risks or side effects must be explained to the patient or a representative of the patient. He or she must agree to the treatment plan before it is started. The agreement is called informed consent, and it is often made official by the patient's signing an informed consent form, which is placed in the medical record.

The documentation content describes the medical care from the moment the patient is admitted to the medical facility to the moment of discharge. The information reporting the effectiveness of the treatment is the content used to determine the quality of the care provided, to measure outcomes and research for the most effective treatment procedures, and to determine reimbursement.

The documentation content is found in the written evaluation reports and the progress notes. The PT performs and writes initial, interim, and discharge evaluations. The PTA can assist the PT in performing the evaluation, but does not write the evaluation. The PTA documents the progress notes. The focus of this text is on writing the progress note.

An overview of these content areas was presented. A more detailed study of each area is presented in Chapters 5, 6, 7, and 8.

REFERENCES   1. Guccione, A: Physical therapy diagnosis and the relationship between impairments and function. Phys Ther 71:499, 1991.
2. Harris, BA: Building documentation using a clinical decision-making model. In Stewart, DL, and Abeln, SH (eds): Documenting Functional Outcomes in Physical Therapy. Mosby–Year Book, St. Louis, MO, 1993, p 83.
3. Goodman, CC, and Snyder, TEK: Differential Diagnosis in Physical Therapy. WB Saunders, Philadelphia, PA, 1990, p 2.
4. Sahrmann, SA: Diagnosis by the physical therapist—a prerequisite for treatment. Phys Ther 68:1703, 1988.
5. Task Force on Standards for Measurement in Physical Therapy: Standards for tests and measurement in physical therapy practice. Phys Ther 71:589, 1991.
6. American Physical Therapy Association: Guidelines for Physical Therapy Documentation. APTA, Alexandria, VA, 1995.

REVIEW EXERCISES

1. List the six categories of documentation content, and describe the content of each category.

2. Explain the difference between subjective and objective data.

3. Define signs and symptoms.

4. Compare and contrast the medical diagnosis and the physical therapy problem.

5. Explain PT and PTA documentation responsibilities.

6. Describe the three types of PT evaluations and how the PTA is involved.

7. Discuss discharge summary versus discharge evaluation.

You read in the PT initial evaluation that your patient has a fractured right femur that has healed. He is left with 2/5 strength in quadriceps and is unable to transfer independently in and out of bed or a chair.

What is the medical problem? _____

What is the PT musculoskeletal problem? _____

What is the functional limitation? _____

In the past, how would the treatment results have been documented?

_____

_____

_____

How should treatment results be documented?

_____

_____

_____

You read in the PT evaluation that your patient has had a CVA (stroke) and now has difficulty moving his left arm and leg. The PT states that the patient has weakness and extensor hyper-tonus in his left lower extremity with inability to ambulate stairs independently.

What is the medical diagnosis? _____

What is the PT neuromusculoskeletal problem? _____

What is the functional limitation? _____

How should treatment results be documented?

_____

_____

_____

You read in the PT evaluation that your patient has an incomplete spinal cord injury causing lower extremity paraparesis and inability to stand.

What is the medical diagnosis? _____

What is the neuromusculoskeletal PT problem? _____

What is the functional limitation? _____

How should treatment results be documented?

_____

_____

_____

Identify the documentation responsibilities of the PT and the PTA. Place "PT" next to the items that are a responsibility of the PT *only*. Place "PTA" next to items that are documentation tasks for the PTA.

_____ Initial evaluation

_____ Progress notes

_____ Measurement results

_____ Progress evaluation

_____ Change in treatment plan

_____ Discharge summary with no interpretation or recommendations

_____ Discharge evaluation

Identify the pathology, impairment, functional limitation, and disability after each patient description.

1. Mr. Jones, a professional football player, will never be able to play football again because he fractured a vertebra and severed his spinal cord. His legs are paralyzed, and he cannot stand or walk.

Pathology _____

Impairment _____

Functional limitation (Nagi)/disability (ICIDH) _____

Disability (Nagi)/handicap (ICIDH) _____

2. Sally received third-degree burns on both hands, and the scar tissue causes limited ROM in her fingers and wrists. She is unable to pick up or manipulate small objects, so she is unable to return to any work that requires fine hand manipulation.

Pathology _____

Impairment _____

Functional limitation (Nagi)/disability (ICIDH) _____

Disability (Nagi)/handicap (ICIDH) _____

3. Mrs. Williams has rheumatoid arthritis with limited ROM in both knees and hips. She is unable to climb stairs or steps, so she must live and function in an environment that has no stairs or steps.

Pathology _____

Impairment _____

Functional limitation (Nagi)/disability (ICIDH) _____

Disability (Nagi)/handicap (ICIDH) _____

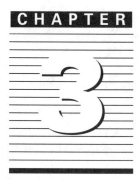

Organization and Presentation of the Content

Learning Objectives:

After studying this chapter, the student will be able to:

■ Find information in the medical record by understanding the organization of the medical record content

■ Organize information to be documented in a physical therapy note into a logical sequence

■ Adapt the information sequencing to a variety of documentation models

■ Use a variety of formats for presentation of the content

■ Understand the PTA's role in Medicare documentation

Information in the medical record **communicates** the story of a patient's medical care. How the information is organized in the chart and the format in which the information is documented varies from facility to facility. How the chart looks depends on the type of clinical facility. The hospital medical record is different from the record in a physical therapy private practice office. The student PTA on internship or the newly employed PTA should immediately become familiar with his or her facility's medical record. It is a good communication tool *only* if the reader knows where to find the information.

ORGANIZATION OF THE MEDICAL RECORD

Until the 1970s, hospitals typically used the **source-oriented** method for organizing the medical record. In the 1970s, the **problem-oriented** method was introduced, offering another method of organizing the medical information. The PTA who has the opportunity to gain work experience in several different clinical facilities may see both types of charts, but will more likely see charts using variations and combinations of source-oriented and problem-oriented organization. In the 21st century, the PTA may be recording in medical records organized according to the **functional** abilities of the patient.

SOMR

The source-oriented medical record (SOMR) is organized according to the medical services offered in the clinical facility. Each discipline has a section in the chart that is labeled with a tab marker or is color coded. The SOMR might be organized with the physician's section first, followed by sections for nursing, physical therapy, occupational therapy, and test results, to name a few. Caregivers in each discipline document their content (data, problems, treatment plans, goals, progress notes, treatment effectiveness) in the section designated for their discipline. The sections must be clearly marked for easy identification so that the reader can locate the information. A criticism of the source-oriented organization is the time required to read through each section for information, making the record difficult to audit for reimbursement and quality control.

Each caregiver on the medical team should be responsible for reading the chart frequently, communicating with the other caregivers, and staying informed as to the patient's latest treatments and condition. One discipline might identify a patient's problem and begin treatment, while the rest of the disciplines may not be aware the problem exists. For example, a nurse discovers high blood pressure and obtains medication orders from the physician. The nurse records this information in the section for nursing notes. The patient experiences side effects from this new medication that affect his ability to understand fully the PTA's exercise instructions. The PTA may not have taken the time to read the nursing section of the patient's chart and is unaware of the addition of this medication. This lack of awareness causes the PTA to make the incorrect assumption that the patient is being uncooperative today, and she records this in the physical therapy section.

To accomplish communication and coordination among the caregivers, regular meetings should be held so that medical personnel can gather to discuss the patient's problems and treatment progress. A written record of the proceedings of the conferences should be placed in the patient's chart.

POMR

In the 1970s, Dr. Lawrence Weed introduced the problem-oriented medical record (POMR). The content in this medical record is organized around the identification and treatment of the patient's problems. The components or sections of the POMR are the (1) data base, (2) problem list, (3) treatment plans, (4) progress notes, and (5) discharge notes. The sections are organized in this order to sequence the information about the patient's medical care from admission to discharge. Each section contains the appropriate information from each discipline. For example, the data gathered by the physician, PT, and occupational therapist (OT) are recorded in the data base section. For each of these disciplines, the problems identified are listed in the problem list section, the treatment plans in the treatment plan section, and the progress notes in the progress note section. Each caregiver may record on the same page within each section, or there may be subsections designated for each discipline within the main sections of the POMR.

POMR was developed by Dr. Weed to eliminate the disadvantages he felt were presented by the SOMR. Communication among disciplines is enhanced because it is easy to read about the problems the other disciplines are identifying and treating. The organization allows specific information, such as the treatment results, to be found easily if the record were audited.

ORGANIZATION OF THE DOCUMENTATION CONTENT

Clinical facilities will differ as to how they organize or sequence the documentation content within the evaluation reports and progress notes. A study of some examples of content organization models reveals a common logic to the sequencing of the information.

SOAP Organization   Presently, the most commonly used method to organize the information is the SOAP organization, developed by Dr. Weed as a component of the POMR. The SOAP writing format (SOAP is a mnemonic for **S**ubjective, **O**bjective, **A**ssessment, **P**lan) organizes the information into a logical sequence and places it in an outline form so that it can be read quickly and easily. It is helpful to "think SOAP" before writing a progress note, no matter what type of format is used. Use of this mnemonic organizes the content into subjective, objective, assessment, and plan categories.

Subjective   S stands for subjective. This section contains the **subjective data**. The S section contains the information *provided by* the patient, his or her caregiver, a family member, or significant other. Each time the patient is seen, he or she is interviewed and questioned. This information is gathered, and the **symptoms** of the patient's disease or dysfunction are described in the subjective section.

Objective   O stands for objective. This section contains the **objective data**. These data must be able to be reproduced or confirmed by another professional with the same training as the person gathering the objective information. This information is gathered by measurable and reproducible tests. It may be obtained through observation and must be described in terms of **functional** movement or actions. The **signs** of the patient's disease or dysfunction are recorded in the objective section. This summary section should "paint a picture" of the patient.

Assessment   A stands for assessment. In this section, the PT or PTA summarizes the S and O information and answers the question "So what?" In the assessment content of the physical therapy evaluation, the PT interprets, makes a clinical judgment, and sets **goals** based on the information in the subjective and objective sections. In the progress note, the PTA summarizes the information in the S and O sections and reports the progress being made toward accomplishing the goals. This summary also answers the "so what?" question.

Plan   P stands for plan. This information describes what will happen next. In the evaluation, the PT's **treatment plan** is outlined in this section. In the progress note, the PTA describes what he or she may need to do before the next treatment session and during the next session.

Examples of SOAP Organization   Suppose your 10-year-old daughter has been diagnosed by your doctor as having strep throat and an ear infection. You obtained medication and have started her on the treatment. It is the next morning.

> **5-18-90**   **Dx/Problem:** Strep throat and ear infection.
>
> ---
>
> **S:**   Pt. reports pain in R ear, feels too tired to go to school.
>
> **O:**   Temperature 100°F, down 2° from last night, skin color pale. Pt. sat at breakfast table 20 min before needing to lie down. Pt. took medication, 2 tablets, 8:00 AM per instructions. _____
>
> **A:**   Pt.'s fever decreasing but temp. not at goal of 98.6°. Pt. is not able to stay up all day for school. _____
>
> **P:**   Will call attendance office to excuse pt. from school, will continue medication per Dr.'s orders.
>
> —Super Parent, PTA

Another example. You are a PTA teaching a patient to walk with crutches. This patient had a skiing accident that resulted in multiple fractures of bones in the ankle joint. The ankle has been surgically treated and casted, and now the patient is not permitted to bear weight on the foot.

2-16-93:   **Dx:** Fractured L ankle, repaired and casted.

Pr: No weight bearing on L requiring ambulation with crutches.

S: Patient states he plans to go home tomorrow and needs to climb a flight of stairs in his house and manage ramps and curbs to return to work.

O: After 3 trials requiring standby assist for sense of security and verbal cuing, patient independently ascended and descended a flight of 12 stairs using the railing (up on R, down on L) and axillary crutches, NWB on L, and independently managed a ramp, and 4 curbs of various heights. Patient independently transferred in and out of his car, accurately following instructions.

A: Patient accomplished his goal of being able to independently manage stairs, ramps, and curbs for functioning within his house and community ambulation for return to work. Patient is ready for discharge.

P: Will arrange for PT discharge evaluation tomorrow.

—Alice Assistant, PTA

You can see how thinking SOAP organizes information so it can be documented in a sequential and logical order. This organization makes finding information an easy task.

Criticism of SOAP   Critics of SOAP format state that the information focuses on the patient's neuromusculoskeletal problems and implies that improvement in these problems will improve the patient's functional abilities. When Dr. Weed introduced the POMR and the SOAP format, documentation content did focus on the impairments (see Chapter 2). Although a SOAP-organized note can be written about functional outcomes, as seen in the crutchwalking example above, a variety of other formats are suggested that are designed with a clearer focus on functional goals.

PSP and PSPG   A format more typically used for the progress note or interim evaluation is the PSP (mnemonic for **P**roblem, **S**tatus, **P**lan), a variation of the SOAP format. First the patient's physical therapy problem and/or medical diagnosis is stated under **P.** The subjective and objective data about the patient's condition at the time of the interim evaluation are documented under **S.** The second **P** is the section that contains the modified treatment plan indicated by the clinical findings. The PSPG format adds the functional goals. Figures 3–1 and 3–2 are examples of notes in PSP and PSPG organization.[1]

ABC Physical Therapy Clinic, Anytown, USA

June 1, 199X

P: 47 YOM, college math professor, Dx: chronic LBP syndrome; mild L spine DJD; probable lumbar extension dysfunction; r/o HNP.

S: Pt. states, "I feel 50% better. The pain in my R leg is gone now. I can sit for over an hour w/o any pain." Pt. attended back school on May 15, 199X. Exam: GMT/AROM WNL, BLE, FAROM, L spine, w/o any c/o Sx. Neg. spasm, TTP, deformity. Neg. SLR to 85° B, neg. Fabere. Gait, posture, SLT WNL. Performs extension exercises w/o difficulty or Sx.

P: Cont w/MH PRN, tid extension exercises, 10–15 reps. F/U w/ Dr. Brown scheduled for tomorrow. PT F/U 2–3 weeks or PRN. Pt. understands home program; pt. questions about exercise techniques answered. _____

—————————————————————————————— Ron Therapist, PT

FIGURE 3–1   A note written in PSP organization. (From Scott, RW: Legal Aspects of Documenting Patient Care. Aspen, Gaithersburg, MD, 1994, p 79, with permission.)

Multidisciplinary Rehabilitation Center, Anytown, USA

June 1, 199X

P: 47 YOM, college math professor, Dx: chronic LBP syndrome; mild L spine DJD; probable lumbar extension dysfunction; r/o HNP.

S: Pt. was discharged as inpatient on May 5, 199X, and placed on OP home PT program of MH PRN and active extension exercises, tid X 10–15 reps. Today pt. states, "I feel 50% better. The pain in my R leg is gone. I can sit for over an hour w/o any pain." Pt. attended back school as inpatient on May 3, 199X. Exam: GMT/AROM WNL, BLE. FAROM, L spine, w/o any c/o Sx. Neg. spasm, TTP, deformity, Neg. SLR to 85°B, neg. Fabere, Gait, posture, SLT WNL. Performs extension exercises w/o difficulty or Sx.

P: Cont. w/MH PRN, tid extension exercises, 10–15 reps. F/U w/Dr. Brown scheduled for tomorrow. PT F/U 2–3 wks or PRN. Pt. understands home program; pt. questions about exercise techniques answered.

G: Decrease residual Sx 50% X 2–3 wks; Ⓘ pain-free ADL; prevent recurrence through good body mechanics._____

———————————————————————————————————— Ron Therapist, PT

FIGURE 3–2   A note written in PSPG organization. This is a physical therapist's 4-week outpatient re-evaluation form. (From Scott, RW: Legal Aspects of Documenting Patient Care. Aspen, Gaithersburg, MD, 1994, p 79, with permission.)

DEP   Another method for organizing and documenting information is the DEP model for performance-based documentation, designed by Smith and El-Din.[2] This mnemonic stands for **D**ata, **E**valuation, **P**erformance goals. The subjective and objective data (**D**) are combined into one section. The evaluation section (**E**) is the interpretation of the data and the identification of the physical therapy problems; the treatment plan is included in this section. The performance goals (**P**) section contains the functional goals toward which the treatment is aimed and the time frame in which the goals are expected to be met.

FOR   Swanson[3] proposed the use of the functional outcome report (FOR), a structured approach for reporting functional assessment and outcomes (Table 3–1). The sequence of the information in the FOR is as follows: (1) reason for referral, (2) functional limitations, (3) physical therapy assessment, (4) therapy problems, (5) functional outcome goals, and (6) treatment plan and rationale. The reason for referral section includes the medical diagnosis, past medical history, and the subjective data. The functional limitations and physical therapy assessment sections contain the objective data. The physical problems are identified based on the data. The functional goals are listed, and the report concludes with the treatment plan and how it will relate to accomplishing the functional goals.

Common Logic for Sequencing the Content   All of these content organization models use a problem-solving approach to sequencing the information. First, the data are gathered. Second, the data are interpreted and a judgment is made as to the identification of the physical therapy problem. Next, goals are set that determine the direction in which the physical therapy care will be aimed. Finally, treatment plans designed to accomplish the goals are outlined. Figure 3–3 is a chart that visually compares the organization models, how they incorporate the documentation content, and how they are similar in their organization.

Guidelines for Adapting to the Organization Varieties   The PTA can easily adapt to any format of documentation when he or she also uses the following problem-solving approach to sequence the information for the progress note:

1. Introduce the progress note with a listing or statement that tells the reader the physical therapy problem(s) about which the note is written.
2. Place the subjective and objective data first. Compare it or relate it to the data in the evaluation.
3. Discuss the meaning of the data as it relates to treatment effectiveness and progress toward accomplishing the functional goals listed in the evaluation.
4. Discuss the plan for future treatment sessions and involvement of the PT.

TABLE 3–1. Example of an Initial Functional Outcome Report

REASON FOR REFERRAL

Patient post meniscectomy of left knee reports pain, stiffness, and difficulty with walking and other upright mobility activities

FUNCTIONAL LIMITATIONS

Activity	Current Status
Sit-to-stand transfer	Independent
Standing balance	Performs independently, with cane
Flat terrain ambulation (speed)	
Flat terrain ambulation (endurance)	Performs with cane for more than 18 sec for 20 ft
	Tolerates less than 5 min
Ambulation on uneven terrain	Unable
Stair climbing	Ascends two steps, descends two steps with railing and minimum assistance

PT ASSESSMENT

Medical diagnosis status post meniscectomy is further defined to include residual left knee joint inflammation

Positive test findings: Positive fluctuation test; limited strength; quadriceps 3/5 and hamstring 4/5, indicative of synovial effusion

THERAPY PROBLEMS

1. Pain on compression maneuvers of the left knee: sitting, sit to stance, periodically during gait cycle, during all phases of stair climbing
2. Difficulty in coordinating gait cycle with use of cane to reduce stress to left knee

FUNCTIONAL OUTCOME GOALS

Activity	Performance	Due date
Flat terrain ambulation (speed)	Independent without device; 20 ft in 9 sec	Within 14 days
Flat terrain ambulation (endurance)	Tolerates unassisted walking for 30 min	Within 21 days
Uneven terrain ambulation	Tolerates for a minimum of 15 min	Within 14 days
Stair climbing	Ascends and descends 15 steps	Within 21 days

TREATMENT PLAN WITH RATIONALE

Application of anti-inflammatory modalities with instruction for follow-up home program to minimize post-activity edema

Lower extremity strength training with instruction in progressive home exercise program

Patient instructed in activity limits and restrictions during the course of care

From Swanson, G: Functional outcome report: The next generation in physical therapy reporting. In Stewart, D, and Abeln, S (eds): Documenting Functional Outcomes in Physical Therapy. Mosby–Year Book, St. Louis, 1993.

This organization is illustrated in the following progress note about the student injured in the motorcycle accident (see Chapter 2):

6-27-93:   **Dx:** Status post pinned fractured R femur.

Pr: Dependent ambulation due to NWB on R leg.

Patient states he feels dizzy when he sits up but is eager to start walking on crutches and go home. Pt. c/o dizziness first time standing during treatment. Blood pressure before treatment 120/70 mmHg, first time up in // bars 108/65 mmHg, second standing trial 118/70 mmHg, after treatment 128/72 mmHg. Pt. ambulated with axillary crutches/minimal assist for sense of security and verbal cues for posture and heel contact/NWB on R/swing through gait 100 ft 2 × in hall, bed ↔ bathroom, and on carpet. Able to Ⓘ sit ↔ stand with crutches from bed/lounge chair/toilet. Pt.'s progress toward goal of Ⓘ community ambulation with crutches 50%. Blood pressure adjusting to upright position. Will teach stairs, ambulation on grass, and car transfers tomorrow AM. Will notify PT discharge evaluation scheduled for tomorrow PM.

—Connie Competent, PTA Lic. #7890

Documentation Content	SOAP	DEP	PSPG	Functional Outcome Report (FOR)
Problem	Pr	D	P	Current therapy problems
Subjective Data	S	D	S	Functional limitations Current status
Objective Data	O	D	S	"
Treatment Effectiveness	A	E	S	"
Goals	A	P	G	Functional outcome goals
Plan	P	E	P	Treatment plan with rationale

FIGURE 3–3   A chart comparing the organization models—how they incorporate the documentation contents and are similar in organization. A = assessment, D = data, E = evaluation, G = goals, O = objective data, P = plan in SOAP and performance in DEP, Pr = problem, S = subjective data in SOAP and status in PPG.

FORMATS FOR THE PRESENTATION OF THE CONTENT

The recording of the information can be done in a variety of formats. Evaluations and progress notes may be handwritten or dictated and typed. The progress notes may be narrative, meaning written in paragraph form, or written in an outline format such as the SOAP note.

Computerized Documentation

Computer software programs are available that are designed for writing evaluations and progress notes. It is possible now to have a computer terminal in every hospital room or in all the treatment areas in a physical therapy department so that the PTA can enter information in the patient's chart immediately after the treatment. Physical therapy documentation software are advertised in publications such as *Physical Therapy* and *PT* magazine.

Flow Charts and Checklists

Much of the data can be recorded on flow charts, fill-in-the blank forms, and checklists. Vital signs, physical therapy modalities used, and functional status of the patient are examples of information that can be listed or checked on a form. Using this format, the caregiver can record in the chart quickly and easily, while the reader can just as easily visually scan the form to gather the information. Hospitals, long-term care facilities, and rehabilitation centers are facilities where the PTA will find narrative or outlined (commonly SOAP) notes, checklists, and flow charts. Figure 3–4 is an example of a flow chart for recording physical therapy treatments. Figure 3–5 illustrates two progress note forms combining checklists and flow charts with brief statements and narration. A fill-in-the-blank form is depicted in Figure 3–6.

Letter Format

Physical therapists in private practice may communicate information about the patient to other caregivers by letter. The data are recorded in the office by any of the models already mentioned, but they are periodically summarized in letter format. This type of format is commonly used when the patient's progress is being reported to a physician.

Individual Educational Program

In the public schools, physical therapy, occupational therapy, speech therapy, and psychological services provided a student are planned and recorded in a format called an **individual educational program** (IEP). This format is in accordance with several laws passed by Congress relating to the provision of services that will facilitate the education of students with disabilities. Professionals representing these services (e.g., teacher, OT, PT, school psychologist, speech pathologist) are included on the IEP team. The team records educational goals and objectives to be accomplished during the school year. The team holds meetings periodically to review the goals and objectives, and it meets with parents a minimum of every 6 months to make any changes that are needed. Table 3–2 lists the components of an IEP. Note how these components are essentially the same components of the physical therapy evaluation and progress note content. Figure 3–7 is an example of the PT's contribution to the annual long-

DATE:						
Orientation/Mood						
UE Strength/Ex	- bicep/tricep					
	- W/C push up/rowing					
	- shld flex/abd/horz abd/add					
TRANSPORT:						
	- transport to dept W/C/cart/amb					
Abductor pillow/knee immobilizer/prothesis/tilt tbl.						
	- standing table					
GAIT:	DEVICE:					
//bars; walker; crutches; cane; Qcane; none						
wt. bearing; NWB; TTWB; PWB; FWB; WBAT						
pattern: 2pt./3pt./4pt.						
distance/endurance						
Balance - sit/stand/walk						
Balance Act: lat/post/braid/line/sit/ball						
Stairs: rail/without rail/gait sequence						
TF's bed mobility						
toilet/raised seat/reg/commode bedside						
slidingboard transfer						
shower seat/car transfers						
supine--> sit; sit --> supine/sit to stand						
EX isometric quad, glut, HS, abd/ball squeeze						
ankle pump/circle/TB DF/PF/Ev/Inv						
hip flexion	supine/sit/stand					
SLR flexion	supine/stand					
SLR extension	prone/stand/side lie					
SLR abduction	supine/side lie/stand					
TKE	supine/sit/SAQ/LAQ					
Bridging	1 leg/both					
knee AAROM	sit/prone/supine					
KA PROM	hip/knee/UE/ankle					
AAROM	hip/knee/UE/ankle					
Stretching	LE/UE					
Positional	ROM/prone/long sit					
CPM						
Modalities	H.P./ice/US/whirlpool					
Neuromusc. Re-Educ. Biofeed/CVA rehab						
HHA/Family instruction in:						
TF's-bed/toilet/shower/chair						
positioning/EX program						
walking program						
Written home program provided						
CHARGE - abbreviation for treatment						
THERAPIST						

SPC 337022   **REHABILITATION PHYSICAL THERAPY**

Restraints: NA / pelvic / vest

DNR Y / N

Precautions:_____

DIAGNOSIS:_____

FIGURE 3–4 Flow chart form for recording physical therapy treatments.

PHYSICAL THERAPY PROGRESS NOTES   HOME CARE / HOSPICE
SERVICES

Patient's Name:	Last		First		Age	Date	Time	Visit Frequency		Date Next Visit

Mood		Orientation		Cooperation		Communication		Pain		RX Tolerance

TREATMENTS			COMMENTS	
Modalities	**WB Status**	**Ambulation**	**Exercise:**	
Bed mobility	Non wt. bearing	Distance		
Elec. stim.	Partial	Assist.		
Ex. active	Toe touch	Balance		
Ex ROM	Full	Coord.		
Ex back	Non amb.	Pattern		
Ex breathing		Stairs		
Ex coord.				
Ex isometric	**Equipment**	**Transfers**	**Problems/Progress:**	
Ex man. resist	Walker	Bed		
Ex mm re-ed.	Crutches	Toilet		
Ex PRE	Cane	Tub		
Ex gait tmg.		Chair		
Massage		Car		
Packs	**ROM**			
Stump wrap				
Transters		Other		
Tx				
Ultrasound				
Evaluation				
MD contact				
Instruction		**Follow-through/Response:**		
Patient				
Support Person				
HHA				

THERAPIST SIGNATURE   7400-17-11/93

FIGURE 3–5   Progress note forms that combine presentation styles. The form on this page combines a checklist with brief statements. The form on the facing page combines a flow chart with narration.

MODALITIES:	DATE/Initials	DATE/Initials	DATE/Initials	DATE/Initials	DATE/Initials	DATE/Initials
Hot Pack/Cold Packs						
Massage/Ice Massage						
Electrical Stimulation						
Traction						
Ultrasound						
Kinetic Activity						
Therapeutic Exercise						
Neuromuscular Re-ed						
Functional Activities						
Training in ADL's						
Serial Casting						
Gait Training						
Orthotics/Prosthetics Train.						
Wound Care						
Whirlpool Therapy						
Conference						
Consultation						
Other						

Date	Comments:

Assessment:

Goals:

Plan:

(Name)	Date	Treatment Diagnosis:
(Name)	Date	
(Name)	Date	

P120 NEW 7/94

Physical Therapy Daily Progress Notes

FIGURE 3–5 Continued.

ACTIVITIES OF DAILY LIVING:

Level of Independence	Without Help	Uses Device	Help of Another	Device & Help	Dependent/ Does Not Do	Not Determined
Feeding						
Hygiene/Grooming						
Transfers						
Homemaking						
Bath/Shower						
Dressing						
Bed Mobility						
Home Mgmt						

Physical Environment: _____

_____

Psychosocial: _____

*Safety Measures: _____

_____

Equipment in Home: _____
Emergency No: _____ *Nutritional Req:_____ Allergies: _____
Unusual Home/Social Environment: _____
*Known Medical Reason Pt. leaves home: _____
Other Services Involved: _____ *Prognosis: _____
Vulnerable Adult Assessment: _____Low Risk _____High Risk
Caregiver Status: _____
Pulse _____ BP _____

Current Medications : _____ _____

_____ _____

_____ _____

Patient's Prior Status: _____

_____

Scheduled MD Follow-up appt (s): _____

_____

Name_____
R# _____

FIGURE 3–6 Form with a fill-in-the-blank format.

TABLE 3–2. Components of an Individualized Educational Program

1. A statement of the student's current levels of educational performance
2. A statement of annual goals, including short-term instructional objectives
3. A statement of the specific special-education and related services to be provided to the student and the extent to which the child will be able to participate in regular education programs
4. The projected dates for initiation of services and the anticipated duration of the services
5. Appropriate objective criteria and evaluation procedures and schedules for determining, on at least an annual basis, whether the short-term instructional objectives are being achieved (34 CFR 300.334).

From American Physical Therapy Association and the Section on Pediatrics: Individualized educational program and individualized family service plan. In Martin, KD (ed): Physical Therapy Practice in Educational Environments: Policies and Guidelines. APTA, Alexandria, VA, 1990, p 6.1.

Learner's Name: _____		
ANNUAL GOALS, SHORT-TERM INSTRUCTIONAL OBJECTIVES		
Thoroughly state the goal. List objectives for the goal, including attainment criteria for each objective.		GOAL# ____ OF _____ GOALS

GOAL:
        The student will independently move about the school building and within the classroom using a wheelchair to participate in all daily school activities, and the student will independently transfer from wheelchair to desk seat, to floor for participation and position change in 6 months.

Short-Term Instructional Objectives

1. The student will independently open doors to the gymnasium and maneuver the wheelchair through the entrance to the gym 1 out of 3 trials in 3 months.

2. The student will independently transfer from wheelchair to floor and back into the chair 1 out of 3 trials in 3 months.

3. The student will safely and independently maneuver the wheelchair around the tables in the cafeteria 1 out of 3 trials in 3 months.

G.   IEP PERIODIC REVIEW

Date Reviewed: _____   Progress made toward this goal and objective

The learner's IEP

☐ Meets learner's current needs and will be continued without changes.

☐ Does not meet learner's current needs and the modifications (not significant) listed below will be made without an IEP meeting unless you contact us.

☐ Does not meet learner's current needs and the significant changes listed below require a revised IEP. We will be in contact soon to schedule a meeting.

NOTE TO PARENT(S): You are entitled to request a meeting to discuss the results of this review.

FIGURE 3–7   An example of the PT's contribution to the goals and instructional objectives on an individual educational program (IEP) written for a child in the school.

DX: R CVA with L hemiplegia INITIAL DATE: 2-24-95

PRECAUTIONS: Broca's Aphasia, feeding tube UPDATE: 3-20-95

Exercise	Set	Rep	Equipment	Assist	Goals
PROM/AAROM L UE & L LE	1	10		muscle belly	1. Independent bed mobility
PRE R UED1 & D2 diagonals, supine	1	10	1# cuff wt	tapping	2. Independent unsupported sitting
	1	10	2# cuff wt	verbal cues	3. Independent wheelchair mobility
	1	as many as he can, goal 10 reps			4. Standing pivot transfer with minimum assist of 1
Resistive active exercise R LE	2	10	2# cuff wt		
SLR, abduction sidelying, prone knee flexion					
TKE long sitting	2	10	1# cuff wt	verbal cues	**TDD:**
Standing 10 min; work on eye tracking and mouth closure			standing table		**TDP:**

Patient's Name	Age	Sex	MD	PT	RM#	Units
Harry A	71	M	Smith	Jones	E123	12

Transfers bed <–> w/c, w/c <–> mat table, w/c <–> toilet, w/c <–> straight chair	Method stand pivot to R side	Assist maximum x1	Other Practice squat pivot transfer w/c <–> mat moving towards L

Pregait/Gait

Stand in // bars - max assist x1 - midline with mirror and wt shifting to L. Watch L knee - no hyperextension.
Sitting balance in w/c with arms removed and in armless straight chair. Minimum assist x2. Work on head movement, eye tracking, wt shifting, trunk rot.
W/c mobility - room to bathroom, room to dining room, to PT department, to OT, speech. Check seating/cushion, L scapula protracted, arm on tray.

FIGURE 3–8 A treatment plan outlined on a cardex, commonly used in physical therapy departments to keep treatment procedures current.

term goals and the instructional objectives in an IEP written for a student. The PTA does not write the physical therapy goals and objectives for the IEP but plays an important role in providing input for their planning. The PTA working in the school environment will document the progress being made toward accomplishing the physical therapy goals.

Cardex

Within the physical therapy department, the patient's treatment goals and current treatment plan may be recorded in a cardex format. This is a 4″ × 6″ card that is kept in a folder designed to hold many cards and be accessed quickly. The information is written in pencil so that it can be updated easily. For example, this morning the card may read that the patient ambulates from his bedroom to the nursing station and ambulates on the carpet in the lounge area. However, during the treatment session later this afternoon, the patient ambulated past the station and to the stairs. The patient also managed three stairs today for the first time. Now the information needs to be erased, and the new ambulation distance and the stair climbing must be described. When the PTA is treating a patient, he or she refers to the cardex information. It is important that the information be updated on a regular basis so that the patient is progressing toward accomplishing the treatment goals. This cardex is to be used within the PT department; it is not a part of the patient's medical record. A treatment plan outlined on a cardex is depicted in Figure 3–8.

Medicare Standardized Forms

Standardized Medicare forms are used to chart the medical care given to patients who have this insurance. The Health Care Financing Administration specifies the format and the time lines in which the data must be recorded and submitted. The Medicare recertification form (Fig. 3–9) is intended to be an evaluation form and should not be completed by a PTA. The approval for physical therapy services is periodically renewed or recertified (at present, every 30 days). When the PT recommends on the form that the therapy be continued for the patient to meet the goals, this becomes an **interim evaluation.** If the patient has reached maximum benefit or has met the goals, this form serves as a **discharge evaluation.** The PTA can pro-

Form Approved
OMB No. 09838-02

PHYSICAL THERAPY
INFORMATION & PLAN OF TREATMENT

(Attach to Medicare Billing Form, continued reimbursement of the treatment program will be based upon the documentation of significant functional improvement of the patients problem or problems.)

| 1 | COVERED X | NONCOVERED ☐ | 2 | CERTIFICATION X | RECERTIFICATION ☐ |

| 3 Patient's Name | Last | First | Middle | 4 Date of Birth | 5 Health Insurance Claim No. |

| 6 Provider Name and Address (City and State) | 7 Provider Number | 8 Attending Physician |

| 9 Admitting Diagnosis ® CVA | 10 Prior Therapy History Dates | 11 Onset 8-1-95 | 12 Date Treatment Started 8/11/95 |

| 13 Rx Diagnosis Same | From None To | 14 Rehab. Potential Good for Goals | 15 Long Range Plan Home with Support |

| 16 Treatment Precautions atri Fib, urinary weakness mild Parkinson. | 17 Functional Status Prior to Current Treatment Episode |

18 Functional Level ☐ = Initial ■ = Last Resort. O = Current Δ = Short Range Goal X = Long Range Goal

Place appropriate symbol on bar.
Unable   Max. Asst.   Mod. Asst.   Minn. Asst.   Sup./Inst.   Indep.

Bed Mobility

Transfers:
- Bed
- Toilet
- Tub/Shower

Ambulation:
- Assistance
- Device   Bars   Walker   Crutches   Quad Cane   SE Cane   None
- Distance Endurance   0'   10   25   100   150   250   300   Times

Other

Skin Integrity   Size ☐ ___   Depth ☐ ___   O ___   Status ___

19 Complicating Factors
- Spasticity ___
- Pain ___
- Contracture ___
- Weakness X
- Balance X
- Motivation ___
- Cognition ___
- Vision/Hearing ___
- Pt. Compliance ___

20 Plans for Continued Therapy:
Yes X   No ___

21 Total No. of Treatmer To Date: 1

22 Treatment Plan:

Exercises to extremities to ↑ strength.
Re-Education to ® ankle
Balance Exercises
Transfers- bed, toilet
gait training- ll bars - progress to walkane - quad cane

Frequency Daily   Duration 3 weeks

23 Remarks:
Pt. had ® CVA with Parapareses
(L). Pt. lives with wife who is supportive + Hopes to return hor
Pt. needs assistance with bed mobility, transfers. He is able
Stand with max ↑ of 1
Quad on L 2/5 Hamstring 1/5
Dorsiflexors - No function.

24 Reason for Terminating Therapy:

25 Certification:
The above plan of treatment is medically necessary and will reasonably treat or diagnose an illness or injury or improve the functioning of a mal-formed body member. The patient is under the care of a physician. This patient was examined by a physician within the past thirty (30) days. Date this examination was _____ . The above plan of treatment was reviewed by me in consultation with the physical therapist on _____ .
(date)

| 26 Physician Signature | Date | 27 P.T. Signature | Date | 28 Therapy Denial or Discharge Date |

F2483 (7/94)   White - Provider; Yellow - Medicare; Pink - Physician; Goldenrod - Provider

FIGURE 3–9   A Medicare recertification form.

vide the PT with information about the status of the patient and can complete the center section with symbols representing the functional level of the patient.

How the information in the medical record is organized depends on the preference of the medical facility. Each facility decides the format in which the data are recorded. The PTA must be familiar with the facility's charting procedures and must always *follow the facility's policies, procedures, and format.*

SUMMARY

Information in the medical chart is organized according to the medical services provided (SOMR), the patient's problems (POMR), or combinations and variations of these two records. Each health care discipline has a section in the SOMR. The POMR sections consist of the data base, problem list, treatment plans, and progress and discharge notes.

The documentation content is organized into a logical sequence: Typically the data are listed first, followed by the interpretation and relevance of the data to the patient's functional abilities and goals and finally the treatment plans. There are a variety of formats for organizing the content, and the PTA must be able to adapt to effectively use the type of format(s) preferred by the facility. The SOAP, DEP, PSPG, and FOR models for content organization were briefly described.

Information in the medical record is recorded in a variety of formats. Notes are written in a narrative paragraph or in a SOAP outline. Flow charts, graphs, checklists, and fill-in-the-blank forms are often used in hospitals and rehabilitation centers, whereas private practice therapists may put the information into a letter to the physician. In schools, the child's treatment plan and goals are incorporated into an IEP. Medicare information is documented on standardized Medicare forms.

REFERENCES

1. Scott, RW: Legal Aspects of Documenting Patient Care. Aspen, Gaithersburg, MD, 1994.
2. El-Din, D, and Smith, GJ: Performance Based Documentation: A Tool for Functional Documentation, Preconference workshop. APTA CSM, February 1995, Reno, NV.
3. Swanson, G: Functional outcome report: The next generation in physical therapy reporting. In Stewart, D, and Abeln, S (eds): Documenting Functional Outcomes in Physical Therapy. Mosby–Year Book, St. Louis, MO, 1993.
4. American Physical Therapy Association and the Section on Pediatrics: Individualized educational program and individualized family service plan. In Martin, KD (ed): Physical Therapy Practice in Educational Environments: Policies and Guidelines. APTA, Alexandria, VA, 1990, p. 6.1.

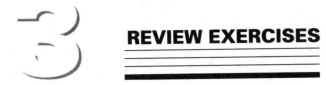

REVIEW EXERCISES

1. Explain how the SOMR and the POMR differ.

2. Describe the information that is documented in each section of a SOAP-organized note.

3. Define PSPG, DEP, and FOR.

4. Discuss how the PTA can adapt to any model for organizing documentation content.

5. List several forms in which documentation content may be presented, and identify the types of physical therapy facilities most likely to use each format.

6. Discuss the PTA role in Medicare recertification documentation.

7. Documentation procedures are different in each physical therapy clinic. What rule should the PTA follow?

Think of two events that occurred recently in your life (e.g., car problem and how you solved it, lost keys and how they were found), and write about them in SOAP format. Organize the information so that **what is told to you** (subjective data) is in the S section, **measurable happenings and things you observed** (objective data) are in the O section, **the meaning of or your conclusions about the data** are in the A section, and **what you plan to do next** is in the P section.

Write one of your notes in outline form using SOAP headings, as in the note on page 28. Write one of the notes in a paragraph form with the information sequenced in SOAP organization, but with no headings.

You have treated your patient and have taken notes about the treatment session. Arrange your notes so that they are in a logical sequence in preparation for writing your progress note. You may want to refer to the guidelines on page 30.

Goal (I) sit to stand met.

Observed patient sitting in middle of couch.

Patient expresses frustration can't get up from couch without help, especially in evening.

Dx: Multiple sclerosis.

Gross MMT 3–/5 all LE muscle groups, 2/5 initial eval.

Pr: LE weakness limiting ability to sit ↔ stand and ambulate safely.

Patient sat at end of couch, scooted forward to edge, used couch arm to help push up. 3rd trial able to sit to stand (I). Verbal cues to lean forward.

Instructed patient not to sit on couch in evening when fatigued and weaker.

Strength gain LEs.

Will visit patient 2 more times and schedule PT discharge evaluation.

Rewrite this unorganized note so the information flows in a logical order. Refer to the guidelines on page 30.

3-26-89

Pt. has met his short-term goal of Ⓘ crutch walking on level and uneven ground. Says he needs to be able to climb three flights of stairs to get to his apartment. Will work on stair climbing next session. Handrail on L going up. Pt. ambulated, NWB R, axillary crutches, Ⓘ, on grass and uneven sidewalk, 300 ft. R ankle & foot edema. Circumference equals L foot & ankle measurements (see initial eval). All R ankle AROM WNL, R knee flexion PROM 10–110° (15–100° last session). Pt. correctly demonstrated self knee ROM & gentle stretching exercises (see copy in chart). RLE mobility progressing. Will inform PT pt. will be ready for discharge evaluation next session. Limited RLE mobility and NWB due to Fx R femur, pinned 3-22-89.

—Confused Student, SPTA/Puzzled Therapist, PT (Lic. #420)

You have been treating your patient who had a R CVA with L hemiplegia, following the treatment plan on the cardex (see Fig. 3–8). Your patient has progressed and the cardex needs to be updated, especially since you will be on vacation next week and another PTA will be seeing your patient. The changes include the following: 5 reps active assistive L scapular protraction in supine with active assistive elbow extension facilitated by tapping triceps muscle belly, RUE PREs 2 lb, 10×/3 lb, 10×/4 lb as many reps as can (stop at 10), 5 lb cuff wts., for all RLE exercises, ambulation in // bars 2× with max. assist of 2 to facilitate wt. shift to L and control knee, using temporary AFO on L ankle, sitting balance now min. assist of 1, now Ⓘ with w/c mobility as brings self to therapy. Standing table discontinued. Other LUE exercises the same.

Write in the changes and update the cardex on the following page.

_DX: _____ INITIAL DATE: _____

_PRECAUTIONS: _____ UPDATE: _____

Exercise	set	rep	equipment	assist	Goals
					TDD:
					TDP:

Patient Name	Age	Sex	MD		PT	RM#	Units

Transfers	Method	Assist	Other

Pregait/Gait

45

You are a PTA working on the orthopedic floor at the local hospital. You are treating Earl, a 62-year-old farmer, who has just had R total knee arthroplasty surgery, and the PT saw him on day 1 postoperation. The discharge goals are (1) independent ambulation on tiling, carpeting, stairs, and inclines with the least restrictive and most appropriate assistive device and (2) independent transfers. Active knee ROM should be 90° at discharge. Treatments are to include CPM, 1 hour on/1 hour off until 70° is reached; isometric exercises for quads, gluts, hamstrings; ankle pumps; TKE; SLR; and active knee flexion. Gait training is to start on day 2 in the AM. A cold pack/ice pack may be used on the knee as needed.

Document the following treatment sessions on the flow sheet on the next page.

Day 2: All isometrics independent with good coordination. CPM increased to 40°. Active knee flexion while supine 3–30°. Bed mobility transfers (supine to sit) mod. assist of one to support knee. Unable to do SLR independently. In sitting, still requires support to R knee as pain too severe for initiation of ROM exercises. Ice pack to knee almost continuous. Drain in place for AM session; removed by PM session. Able to stand at side of bed, PWB RLE. Did not attempt ambulation due to pain.

Day 3: AM: Able to sit at side of bed with AROM to 45°, much pain. BP 140/85 mmHg, pulse at 72 BPM prior to standing. Stood at side of bed with mod. assist of one, PWB to approx. 50% of body weight on RLE, used walker. Took several steps to chair, then sat. Uses standing pivot transfer with walker. BP 145/88 mmHg, pulse 100 BPM. Independent with all exercises. Supine knee flexion to 35°. CPM to 60° PM as in AM, but able to ambulate 50 ft 1× with walker, PWB at 50% body weight. Continues to keep ice pack on knee.

Day 4: AM: Ambulated 50 ft 2× with walker on level surface, tile, and carpet. Sitting AROM 60°, CPM increased to 70°. Supine AROM 5–55° flexion. Min. assist with SLR. PM: ambulated 50 ft 2× with walker, SBA. Ambulated 60 ft 1× with crutches on level, min assist of one. Remains PWB with up to 75% body weight. AROM sitting to 75 degrees, supine 5–60°. SBA for supine to sit transfer, independent transfer sit to stand. Independent with SLR. Ice pack discontinued this morning.

Day 5: AM: Independent with all exercises and all standing pivot transfers. CPM discontinued last night by nursing. Ambulates independently 125 ft with crutches, 3-point step through gait on tile and carpeting. SBA on stairs and inclines. Knee ROM sitting to 85°, supine 5–80°. PT to see patient in PM for discharge evaluation.

TOTAL KNEE ARTHROPLASTY

	Date 8-8-95		Date		Date		Date		Date	
	am	pm	am	pm	am	pm	am	pm	am	pm
CPM Degrees	25	25								
CPM Time	1 hr on/1 hr off									
Knee ROM AA = Active Assist A = Active Supine										
Sitting										
Exercises: Isometrics Quads/Gluts/HS										
Ankle Pumps										
TKE										
SLR										
Active Knee Flex										
Transfers: Bed Mobility										
Toilet/Commode										
Shower Seat										
Car Transfer										
Standing Pivot										
Sliding Board										
Supine <--> Sit										
Sit <--> Stand										
Balance: Sitting										
Standing										
Ambulation: Device										
Weight Bearing										
Pattern										
Distance										
Surface										
Assist										
Stairs										
Blood Pressure										
Pulse										
Modalities	ice pack prn									
THERAPIST	Jennifer Nice, PT									

PHYSICAL THERAPY PROGRESS

PRECAUTIONS: Drain in place 8-8-95

NAME: Earl

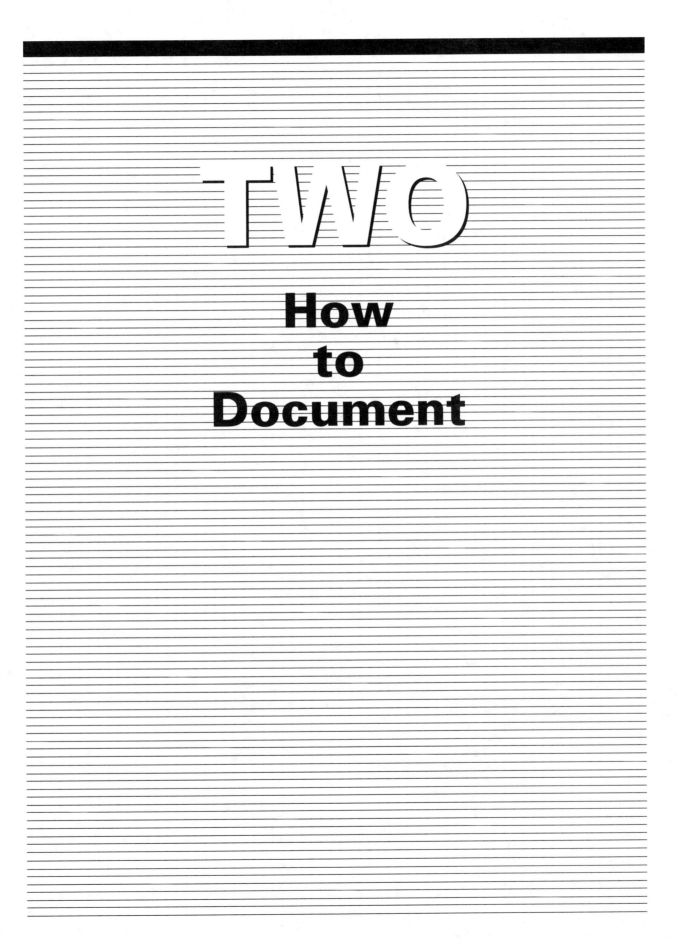

TWO

How
to
Document

Writing the Content: Guidelines

Learning Objectives

After reading this chapter the student will be able to:

- Discuss the use of the progress note in the medical record
- Recognize a variety of formats for presenting the progress note information
- List the guidelines for documenting in a legal record
- Read sample progress notes, and identify what legal guidelines were not followed

The previous three chapters discussed the purpose for documentation, defined documentation, identified the categories of content or information that is documented in the medical record, and presented a variety of formats in which the content may be organized. The next five chapters focus on the actual writing of the content. The guidelines, instructions, and suggestions center around the progress note written by the PTA.

THE PROGRESS NOTE

In the medical record, the progress notes are the **record of the treatment procedures administered.** In the physical therapy chart, they are the written report of the patient's physical therapy treatment sessions. The information is proof that the treatment plan outlined in the initial evaluation is being carried out and that the treatment progression is focused on the accomplishment of the goals determined in the initial evaluation. It is evidence that the treatment procedures are appropriate and effective, providing important information for the purpose of reimbursement and quality assurance.

Writing Frequency

The progress note is written after each treatment session or after a series of sessions. The frequency of the documentation is influenced by the requirements of the insurance company, the documentation standards the facility must follow, and the facility's policies. Typically, the more acute the patient's condition, the more frequently the progress notes are written, and progress notes are documented less frequently with chronic conditions. PTs and PTAs most commonly document daily or weekly.

Content and Form

According to the APTA's *Guidelines for Physical Therapy Documentation*,[1] continuum-of-care documentation should include identification of specific treatments provided; equipment provided; and client status, progress, or regression. The note should state specifically what was done during the treatment session and the functional outcome.

In most facilities the notes are written in either narrative form or SOAP outline. However, the information may be in other similar formats such as the DEP, FOR, or PSPG (see Chapter 3). Many use formats that combine descriptive information with flow sheets, check-off forms, or graphs and charts. Figure 4–1 illustrates a PTA progress note written as a narrative or paragraph. The reader will recognize that the information is *organized* in the SOAP format.

Diagnosis and Problem in the Progress Note

The diagnosis and the problem may introduce the progress note in the medical record, as illustrated in Figures 4–1 and 4–2. Not all facilities use this format, but the PTA may see this in a POMR. When the problems are listed and numbered on the problem list in the POMR, then the number of the problem and/or diagnosis being documented is placed in the margin or at the heading of the note. In many facilities, the problems are not numbered.

> *Example:*
> 1. **Dx:** Multiple sclerosis
>   **Problem #2:** Ataxia of lower extremities
> 2. **Dx:** Fractured right femur
>   **Problem:** 2/5 strength of quadriceps

PRINCIPLES FOR DOCUMENTING IN A LEGAL RECORD

Following the principles and guidelines for documenting in the legal record will provide the PTA with a good start toward quality care and documentation. The guidelines for documenting in the medical record are incorporated into each facility's documentation standards. Again, the best rule is to *follow the facility's procedures*.

Legal Guidelines

Document with the assumption that the information will be read by lawyers and jurists in court. When writing in a medical record, think, "*Dear ladies and gentlemen of the jury*."[2] This will remind the PTA that the medical record is a legal document and, therefore, that guidelines must be followed.

Be Accurate

"*Never* record falsely, exaggerate, or make up data." (p 8).[3] Information that is pertinent to the patient's care should never be omitted, even if it might be damaging to the PTA. The court is more likely to be lenient when all information is recorded in the medical record and a mistake is admitted. Keep information relevant to the patient.

5-18-90 **Dx:** Fx R hip.
        Problem #2: Dependent ambulation 2° Fx R hip.
        Pt. states his hip feels sore today but not painful; feels he should be able to walk better. Pt. ambulated bed to dining room (330 ft) with min. assist 1X for loss of balance recovery 2X, standard walker, partial weight-bearing on right. Posture erect, pt. looks ahead. Quality of pt.'s gait & balance improved (see 5-16-90 note), making good progress toward goal of independent ambulation. Continue ambulation training per PT initial plan. Will teach stair climbing next session and add ambulation on carpet. _____
                                _____ Jane Doe, PTA (Lic. #)

FIGURE 4–1   A PTA progress note is written as a narrative or paragraph, but the information is *organized* in SOAP form.

> 9-12-95 AM **Dx:** L hip fracture.
>   **Problem #6:** Dependent with pivot transfer.
> **S:** Patient states she pivoted chair <---> bed with minimal help from daughter last night. _____
>   9-12-95 ss
> **O:** ~~Instructed pt in~~ After three trials, pt. stood & pivoted non–weight-bearing on left, chair <—>
>   mat, WC <—> toilet, bed <—> WC with SBA for loss of balance recovery if needed. No loss of
>   balance. _____
> **A:** Pt. ready for pivot transfer with SBA with nursing. Making good progress toward goal of independent
>   transfers. _____
> **P:** Will notify PT & nursing.—Sally Student, SPTA/Mary Therapist, PT (Lic. #)

FIGURE 4–2   An example of a progress note following legal guidelines.

Be Brief   State information in short, concise sentences. Keep the note brief by staying focused on the information *relevant* to the effectiveness of the treatment and to changes and improvement in the patient's functional abilities. Abbreviations should be used sparingly and *preferably not at all*. The medical record containing documentation consisting mainly of abbreviations may not accurately **communicate** the patient's care.

ABBREVIATIONS   Medical documentation traditionally has demonstrated an overuse of abbreviations. Each health discipline has a long list of abbreviations for its unique terminology. Individual clinical facilities have their lists of acceptable abbreviations, but the lists may differ somewhat from facility to facility. The use of some abbreviations may be common within a facility, community, or region, but may never be used in other facilities or areas or may be used with different definitions. Table 4–1 lists the medical terms that have the abbreviation PT or PTA. Davis, in *Medical Abbreviations: 10,000 Conveniences at the Expense of Communications and Safety,*[4] writes:

> Abbreviations are sometimes not understood or are interpreted incorrectly. Their use may lengthen the time needed to train individuals in the health fields, at times delays the patient's care and occasionally results in patient harm (p 1).

Davis offers the following example of how the patient's care may be delayed due to the misinterpretation of the abbreviation PT.

> The order for PT, intended to signify a lab test order for prothrombin time, resulted in the ordering of a physical therapy consultation (p 1).

It cannot be assumed that the reader will take the time to look up the meaning of each unfamiliar abbreviation. Payment for the patient's care may be denied if the insurance representative does not understand the abbreviations. The use of abbreviations presents the risk that

TABLE 4–1. List of Medical Terms Abbreviated as PT or PTA

PT	PTA
Cisplatin	Percutaneous transluminal angioplasty
Parathormone	Physical therapy (*sic*) assistant[*]
Parathyroid	Plasma thromboplastin antecedent
Paroxysmal tachycardia	Post traumatic amnesia
Patient	Pretreatment anxiety
Phenytoin	Prior to admission
Phototoxicity	Pure-tone average
Physical therapy	
Pine tar	
Pint	
Posterior tibial	
Preterm	
Prothrombin time	

Davis uses the term "physical therapy assistant," which is incorrect. This mistake is commonly seen. Physical therapy personnel must promote the use of the correct term, "physical *therapist* assistant."
From Davis, NM: Medical Abbreviations: 10,000 Conveniences at the Expense of Communications and Safety, ed 7. Neil M Davis Associates, Huntingdon Valley, PA, 1995, pp 176–177.

the patient may receive inappropriate or even dangerous treatment because an abbreviation was misinterpreted. For example, the PTA would make a serious mistake if the abbreviation TWB was interpreted as *total weight bearing* instead of *touch weight bearing* for a patient with a recent hip fracture!

Although risky, abbreviations are presently being used in documentation. Therefore, the student PTA does need to understand the definitions or abbreviations used in physical therapy and must know where to find the definitions of other abbreviations. Abbreviations have been used in examples and practice exercises in this text. A list of those abbreviations with their definitions is located in Appendix A. Medical terminology and physical therapy documentation texts are additional resources for abbreviation lists.

Be Clear

The **meaning** must be immediately clear to the reader. Use words to paint a picture of the patient's functioning and condition. The description should allow the reader to "see" the patient accurately in the mind's eye. (e.g., In sitting position, client grasps pant's leg to lift and place L lower leg on R knee to reach L shoe.) See Chapter 6 for instructions on how to describe a patient's functioning.

Handwritten documentation must be **legible.** If the handwriting is difficult to read, the information may be interpreted incorrectly. This creates the potential that unsafe or inappropriate treatment will be provided. Payment for treatment may be denied if the insurance representative finds the handwriting too difficult to read. To avoid the problem of poor handwriting, many facilities require that all documentation information be dictated and typed by a medical transcriptionist. Other facilities have computers in the clinic that contain documentation software designed for physical therapy evaluations and notes. Examples of documentation using computer software are in Appendix B, and information about dictating techniques are in Appendix C.

Punctuation, grammar, and spelling must be correct. This demonstrates attention to detail and implies quality work. Spelling errors may suggest to the reader that the caregiver can be careless and thus could make errors in patient care.

Date and Sign All Entries

Documentation *must be signed* with the caregiver's **legal signature** followed by the abbreviation for his or her professional title (e.g., Sally M. Smith, PTA. Lic. #123). Progress notes written by PTAs do not need to be co-signed by a PT. However, some facilities require that either all notes or certain periodic notes written by the PTA be co-signed by the supervising PT, depending on how the facility interprets the criteria set by the insurance company and the state's physical therapy practice act (e.g., Sally M. Smith, PTA/Jane Doe, PT). Notes written by students *must* be co-signed by the supervising PT or PTA (e.g., Joe Citizen, SPTA/Jane Doe, PTA, Lic. #456).

The APTA is recommending that PTs and PTAs include their license or registration number after their title in all documentation.[1] Several other health care providers include some of the same modalities in their treatments as are included in physical therapy treatments (e.g., hot packs, whirlpool, ultrasound, and massage are often administered by chiropractors, athletic trainers, and massage therapists). Audits are performed on medical records to determine whether a modality is being overused or used effectively. The license number identifies that the modality was administered by a physical therapy provider and distinguishes it from modality treatments given by other health care providers.

Every note *must* be dated, and the date should be easy to see. Most commonly the date is located in the left margin at the beginning of the note. Figure 4–3 depicts a progress note properly dated and signed.

Use Black Ink

Use of black ink is a common guideline but subject to change. The PTA should follow the facility's procedure. Black ink traditionally had been used because it copied more clearly than other ink colors. Technology of copying machines has progressed so that other ink colors now copy clearly and appear black. Some lawyers are now having legal documents signed in blue ink so as to distinguish the original from the copy. Other colors such as green, mauve, or taupe may copy well but are not appropriate for a medical record.

> **5-14-90** **Dx:** Multiple sclerosis.
> **Problem #2:** Ataxia of lower extremities.
> Patient stated she fell yesterday when attempting to step up onto a curb; second time this week she has fallen. Bruise on left lower leg observed. Patient attempted to step up onto stool and stubbed toe. Coordination exercises performed with emphasis on foot lifting and placement. Home program provided (see written program in chart). Following exercise session, patient accurately placed foot on stool and stepped up independently. Patient is able to control foot placement with visual cues and concentration. Patient to return on 5-21-90 for follow-up. Check on home exercise program and coordination progress per PT plan. _____
> ——————————————————————————————————— Sue Smith, PTA

FIGURE 4–3 A progress note properly dated and signed.

Do Not Allow Opportunity for the Record to be Changed or Falsified

It should be difficult for someone to change or alter the written note.

Do not use erasable pens.

Do not erase errors. Draw a line through the mistake, date and initial directly above the
error (e.g., patient ambulated with ~~crutches~~ standard walker).
3-4-93 ML

Do not leave empty lines. Empty spaces provide the opportunity for someone to falsify the record by adding to or changing the information. Draw a horizontal line through empty spaces.

Be Timely

Document as soon as possible after seeing the patient, while the information is fresh in your mind. The progress note that is written immediately after the patient treatment session is the most accurate note. It is more likely that the PTA may move from one patient to the next and treat a full day's schedule of patients before being able to document. The PTA should carry a small notebook to take notes *while* treating the patient so that each patient's progress note will be accurate and thorough.

Treatments that are provided twice a day may be documented by placing AM or PM after the date (12-4-93 AM) (12-4-93 PM). This allows another health care provider such as the OT, nurse, or speech pathologist to document in the progress note section of the chart between the physical therapy AM and PM notes, thus illustrating the continuum of care throughout the day. An addendum is made when information is added to a note that has already been written and signed. To add more information later, date the new entry and state "addendum to physical therapy note dated _____."

Figure 4–2 is an example of a progress note that follows legal guidelines.

SUMMARY

The PTA writes the progress note that provides proof that the physical therapy treatment plan is being carried out. It is a record of the patient's progress and the effectiveness of the treatment. The progress note may be written in various formats but is commonly written in narrative paragraph or SOAP outline forms. It is part of a legal record and is written in accordance with guidelines for legal documentation. These guidelines have been listed and described in this chapter.

REFERENCES

1. American Physical Therapy Association: Guidelines for Physical Therapy Documentation. APTA, Alexandria, VA, 1995.
2. Somerness, W: Work Hardening, Specialties in Occupational Medicine. Notes from workshop presentation, August 1986, Superior, Wisconsin.
3. Kettenbach, G: Writing SOAP Notes. FA Davis, Philadelphia, 1995, p 8.
4. Davis, NM: Medical Abbreviations: 10,000 Conveniences at the Expense of Communication and Safety, ed 7. Neil M Davis Associates, Huntingdon Valley, PA, 1995, p 1.

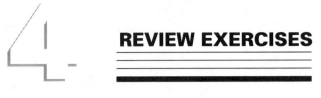

1. Discuss the importance of the progress note to the medical record, the frequency of writing, and who writes it.

2. The progress note information can be presented in a variety of forms. List examples.

3. List the guidelines for writing in a legal record. Explain the purpose of each guideline.

4. Discuss why the use of abbreviations is not recommended.

5. Explain why APTA recommends that PTs and PTAs include their license numbers when signing physical therapy documentation.

You are reading your new patient's chart and you see the progress note written with so many abbreviations that you are not sure you really understand it. Rewrite the note so that it is still as brief as possible, but any reader would understand it. Follow this hospital's SOAP documentation style. Follow guidelines for documenting in a legal record.

9-17-94   **Dx:** L TKA.

Pr: Unable to ambulate Ⓘ, R LE weakness, PWB allowed.

S: Pt wife states he slept "poorly" last two noc. Min c/o pain w/ex during tx session.

O: Pt OOB R w/mod A ×1. Dangled ×5 min w/ c/o dizziness. Gt trng w/fw/w PWB L flat surface × 30 ft ×2 w/5 min rest. Pt ret. to bed for ther ex. to L LE of quad set 10 reps 4 sec hold w/strong contraction. SLR × 10 reps w/ER to 10° lag. AROM L knee 10–50°, PROM 0–60°.

A: ↑ROM, ↑distance. Pt making gains even though N/A to sleep well. Pt. expected to achieve STG of ↑ROM, ↑str, and min A gt.

P: Cont. w/gt trng & ther ex. Begin stair amb. PM 9/18/94. J. T., PTA

_____

_____

_____

_____

_____

_____

_____

_____

_____

List the legal guidelines the PTA did *not* follow when writing the following progress note:

Dx: Psoriasis both arms.

Pr: Difficulty sleeping and concentrating due to severe itching.

S: Pt. states R elbow itches alot. States his knees feel stiff, has trouble getting up out of his favorite chair. He likes to sit in his chair with his cat in his lap and they watch the traffic go by.

O: Seen pt. 4 times. Ultraviolet treatment to both arms to dry up the soars. Rash gone from L forearm.

A: Pt. tolerating treatment OK.

P: Continue per PT initial plan.

_____

_____

_____

_____

_____

List the legal guidelines the PTA did *not* follow when writing the following progress note:

11-17-92   **Dx:** L CVA.

Pr: Weakness in R UE & LE with unsafe ambulation and dependent in ADLs.

      Pt. states not doing exercises at home. Has not been going out to church or club meetings because she is afraid of falling. Pt. states she has always been active and wishes she could go to her brige club meetings. She loves to play brige and misses her brige club friends the most. They have been friends since they were girls together in grade school. L hand extremely purple! Can't bare wt on hand due to stiffness in fingers, decreased ROM in all finger joints. Can't push on hand to get up off of floor. Isometrics to shoulder, lots of cheating. ~~PROM~~ AAROM biceps/triceps, shoulder flexion/extension, shoulder internal rotation/external rotation, forearm pronation/supination, shoulder abduction/adduction, wrist flexion/extension, wrist ulnar deviation/radial deviation, 10 reps each in supine position. Independent supine to sit if role to R elbow for support and push with L hand to get up. Pt has difficulty comprehending: and is impatient: and is uncooperative. Will continue treatment 3×/wk per PT plan. M. Lukan

_____

_____

_____

_____

_____

Rewrite the progress note in Practice Exercise 2 using the correct legal guidelines. This progress note is poorly written, but do not try to improve the content. Correct only the legal guidelines errors. You will be asked to improve the content of this note in a practice exercise later in the text.

_____

_____

_____

_____

_____

_____

_____

_____

Rewrite the progress note in Practice Exercise 3 using the correct legal guidelines. This progress note is poorly written, but do not try to improve the content. Correct only the legal guidelines errors. You will be asked to improve the content of this note in a practice exercise later in the text.

_____

_____

_____

_____

_____

_____

_____

_____

_____

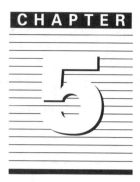
Writing the Content: Subjective Data

Learning Objectives
After studying this chapter, the student will be able to:
- Recognize subjective data information
- Select and document subjective data information that is relevant to the patient's problem and treatment
- Organize subjective data information for easy reading and understanding
- Follow recommended guidelines for documenting subjective data information
- Properly document information about the patient's pain

The **subjective data** content in the physical therapy evaluation report and the progress note is typically located at the beginning of or early in the note, no matter which organizational format is used. It is recorded in the S section of the SOAP outline, in the D section of the DEP format, and in the F section of the FOR. Subjective data content is included in the S (status) section of the PSPG organization. It is important information in the evaluation reports, but it may or may not be necessary in the interim or progress notes. It is necessary only if it provides evidence of treatment effectiveness or progress toward the functional goals.

Subjective data are more important to the health care provider than to the lawyer or insurance representative. The health care provider learns from the patient pertinent and useful information about the patient's condition and the effects of the medical treatment. The lawyer and the third-party payer are interested primarily in the results or outcomes of the medical care.

DEFINITION OF SUBJECTIVE DATA

Subjective data consist of information that the patient, significant other, or caregiver *tells* the PT and PTA and that is *relevant* to the patient's present condition and treatment.

Relevant Information

One of the key words in that definition is **relevant**. A common mistake seen in progress notes is the inclusion of information that does not relate to the patient's problem or the treatment session (Fig. 5–1). It is not easy to confine the subjective information to just relevant information. The PTA and the patient will likely have conversations about a variety of subjects. Important information about the patient's problem often slips out during a seemingly unrelated conversation. The PTA must be an alert listener and sort out the relevant information.

Listening for Relevant Information

Effective listening is a skill that is consciously developed with practice. To sort out the relevant information, the PTA should be aware that much of the work day is spent **listening** in a variety of ways. Some listening techniques are listed as follows:

1. **Analytic listening** for specific kinds of information (e.g., pain, lifestyle, fears)
2. **Directed listening** to a patient's answers to specific questions (e.g., What positions increase frequency or intensity of pain? What does the patient need to be able to do at work?)
3. **Attentive listening** for general information to get the total picture of the patient's situation
4. **Exploratory listening** because of one's own interest in the subject
5. **Appreciative listening** for aesthetic pleasure (e.g., listening to music on headphones while walking during lunch break)
6. **Courteous listening** because it is the polite thing to do
7. **Passive listening** by overhearing (e.g., conversation in the next treatment booth)

Analytic, directed, and attentive listening provide information that may be relevant for subjective data content in the progress note. More relevant information may be revealed when exploratory listening is used.

Examples of Relevant Information

The PTA should be familiar with the patient's medical record and should have read the PT's initial evaluation as well as the initial evaluations of the physician and any other health care providers treating the patient. During treatment sessions, the PTA should listen for any information that relates to treatment effectiveness and accomplishment of goals. The PTA should report to the PT and document in the progress note any information he or she hears that is not in the record, but important for effective and quality physical therapy care of the patient.

MEDICAL HISTORY

> **Initial Evaluation:** Information about the patient's previous medical conditions and treatments are in the medical history section of the medical chart and in the initial evaluations.
> **Progress Note:** Listen for any medical history information that was not reported earlier but is relevant to the patient's treatment.

11-17-92 **Dx:** L CVA.
　　　　　Pr: Weakness in RUE & LE with unsafe ambulation and dependent in ADLs.
　　　　　Pt. states not doing exercises at home; has not been going out to church or club meetings because she is afraid of falling. Pt. states she has always been active and wishes she could go to her bridge club meetings. She loves to play bridge and misses her bridge club friends the most. They have been friends since they were girls together in grade school. They just celebrated their 65th year of friendship! _____

_____

_____ Robert Relevant, SPTA/ Tom Jones, PTA

FIGURE 5–1 Subjective data section of a progress note containing superfluous information.

Example: Sue, the PTA, sneezes four times as she escorts Mrs. Smith to the treatment cubicle to prepare for an ultrasound treatment. As she excuses herself to go wash her hands, Sue explains that she is not sick but is allergic to pollen during this time of the year. Mrs. Smith mentions her allergy to a perfume that Sue knows is in the ultrasound gel. As Sue positions Mrs. Smith on the plinth, Mrs. Smith states that she itched for awhile "right where the PT gave my first ultrasound treatment yesterday." Sue makes a mental note to use ultrasound lotion instead of the gel today, to tell the PT, and to be sure to document this in the progress note. Figure 5–2 demonstrates how this information is included in the progress note.

ENVIRONMENT: LIFESTYLE, HOME SITUATION, WORK TASKS, SCHOOL NEEDS, LEISURE ACTIVITIES

Initial Evaluation: The PT already will have interviewed the patient to learn about his or her needs at home to help plan treatment goals.

Progress Note: Listen for any further information that will influence treatment.

Example: Sue knows from reading the medical record that her patient, Harry, has a combination tub and shower with grab bars at home, his bathroom is small, and the toilet is next to the tub. Harry had a stroke, and his balance is slightly unsteady. Sue is planning to teach him to slide from the toilet onto the edge of the tub, to swing his feet into the tub, then to stand for his shower. Today, during his treatment session, Harry's wife comments that her back is aching because she just spent an hour cleaning the shower doors and the track in which the doors slide. "That track is uncomfortable to sit on," thought Sue. "I need to think of a better method for Harry to transfer into his tub."

EMOTIONS OR ATTITUDES

Initial Evaluation: The PT records the patient's attitude or emotional state presented at the time of the evaluation.

Progress Note: Patient's attitudes can change during the course of treatment, or they might not have presented their true feelings to the PT during the initial evaluation. The PTA should be alert for these changes.

Example: PTA Jim treats his patient Sam, who had a stroke. Yesterday, they worked on balance and stability using the hands-and-knees position and batting a balloon while in sitting position. Today Sam refuses to go to physical therapy. He states that he does not want to play children's games and that if he could just go home, he would be fine. Jim

---

4-19-94 Pr: Subdeltoid bursitis with decreased deltoid strength and decreased shoulder ROM interfering with ability to perform work tasks.

S: Pt. reports itching "right where the PT gave my first ultrasound treatment yesterday." Mentioned she is allergic to some perfumes.

O: No skin rash or redness observable in treatment area today. Direct contact US/1 MHz/1.5 w/cm^2 (moderate heat)/5 min/R subdeltoid bursa/sitting/shoulder extended/arm resting on pillow to decrease inflammation. Used ultrasound lotion instead of gel. Gel contains perfume. Pt. correctly performed home exercise program of isometrics for the deltoid, holding for 8 counts (see copy in chart).

Shoulder AROM:	before tx	after tx
flexion	0–55°	0–60°
abduction	0–68°	0–73°

A: Treatment tissue less sensitive to US (1 w/cm^2 yesterday). US effective in reducing inflammation. Pt. beginning to progress toward goal of decreased inflammation, improved shoulder mobility to perform work tasks.

P: Will monitor pt.'s response to the US lotion tomorrow and alert PT of the reaction to the gel. Pt. is scheduled for four more treatments.—Sue Citizen, PTA

FIGURE 5–2 Adding new relevant subjective information to the medical record through the progress note.

realizes he needs to consult the PT and restructure the treatment sessions to work on balance and stability in activities Sam will want to be doing at home.

GOALS OR FUNCTIONAL OUTCOMES

Initial Evaluation: Goals or functional outcomes are set by the patient and the PT during the initial evaluation.

Progress Note: Goals may need to be modified as the patient and the PTA become better acquainted and the PTA learns more about the patient's needs and desires.

Example: Sam told the PT that he only needs to be able to climb two steps to get into his house; the rest of his house is on one floor. They set a stair-climbing goal: "To be able to climb two steps independently using railing on the left and to be able to ascend and descend a curb independently with no ambulation device." One week later, during a treatment session, Sam is telling Jim about his cabin on a nearby lake and how anxious he is to go to the cabin and go fishing. Sam casually mentions that there are six wooden steps down to the dock. Jim makes a mental note to share this information with the PT and to suggest that the goal be modified.

UNUSUAL EVENTS OR CHIEF COMPLAINTS

Initial Evaluation: Chief complaints are the patient's **symptoms** of the disease or dysfunction requiring treatment.

Progress Note: During treatment sessions, reports of unusual events may indicate a physiologic change in the patient, or may be evidence of the effectiveness or ineffectiveness of the treatment. Reports may also indicate the patient's compliance and/or other health conditions during the week.

Example 1: Patient states she did not do her home exercises this week because she had the flu.

Example 2: PTA Brenda treats Ray, who has a spinal cord injury. Today she goes to Ray's hospital room to take him to physical therapy. Ray complains he is feeling weak, has chills, and is somewhat light-headed. He doesn't think he can exercise in therapy today. Brenda talks with Ray's nurse and cancels this morning's therapy. Brenda checks on Ray in the afternoon, and he tells her that he has a urinary tract infection and is just now starting the medication. He still feels weak and light-headed. Brenda cancels the afternoon treatment session.

RESPONSE TO TREATMENT

Progress Note: This documents the effectiveness of treatment and influences future treatment plans.

Example: PTA Brenda treats Robert who has a mild lumbar disc protrusion and who complains of waking up often in the night with tingling in his left leg. During yesterday's treatment session, Brenda showed Robert how to use pillows and a rolled towel to support his spine and to maintain proper positioning while sleeping. Today, Robert reports that he only awoke three times last night because of back soreness and that he did not have any tingling in his leg.

LEVEL OF FUNCTIONING

Initial Evaluation: This describes the patient's functional level at the time of the evaluation.

Progress Note: The patient may describe a functional level that could be a way of measuring his or her progress or response to treatment.

Example: PTA Mary is treating Mr. Jones, who had an acute flare-up of osteoarthritis in his hands. His chief complaint during the initial evaluation was inability to dress himself, especially handling buttons and snaps, because of the pain. Today he arrives wearing a sweater, which he said he buttoned without needing to ask for help.

> Pt. c/o pain in R shoulder when R arm is hanging down. Lives alone. Pt.'s goal is to play on the college volleyball team this winter. Denies having previous injury or trauma to shoulder. C/o pain when attempting to put on sweater and T-shirts. States he is limited to only a few clothing items he can get into without help. States his shoulder started to ache for no apparent reason. Has been practicing volleyball 6 hr/day for the last 3 weeks.

FIGURE 5–3 Documentation that randomly presents subjective data, making it difficult to get a clear picture of patient's status.

ORGANIZING AND WRITING THE SUBJECTIVE CONTENT

Organizing the Subjective Data

The subjective content in the initial evaluation may be more complex and detailed than the subjective information in the progress note. The PT may organize this information into subcategories such as complaints (c/o), history (Hx), environment, and pt.'s goals or functional outcomes, behavior, and description of pain. This helps the PT to confine the data to only the categories that are relevant. Organizing the content makes it easy to read and locate information. The example in Figure 5–3 randomly presents subjective data, making it difficult to get a clear picture of the patient's status. In Figure 5–4, the note is rewritten, with the information grouped according to topic.

The PTA needs to document subjective data *only* if there is an update of the previous information or if there is relevant new information. Usually the content is brief. If the information is about more than one topic category, it should be grouped according to the topics, but it may not be necessary to identify the topic categories. Instances when progress notes may not contain subjective information are when relevant information was not provided or when the patient was unable to communicate (e.g., patient in a coma) and there was no one else present during the treatment to offer subjective data.

Guidelines for Writing the Subjective Data

Verbs

When documenting the subjective data, use verbs that make it clear to the reader that the information is being provided by the patient. Use verbs such as *states, reports, complains of, expresses, describes, denies.* It is not necessary to repeat the word "patient" (or pt.) After it is used once, it is assumed that all the information in the section was told by the patient, as in the examples in Figure 5–5.

Quoting the Patient

Occasionally it is better to quote the patient directly, rather than paraphrasing the patient's comments. Quoting will make the intent of the comment or the relevance to the treatment clearer. The following are good situations in which to quote the patient:

1. To illustrate **confusion** or **loss of memory.** (*Example:* Pt. often states, "My mother is coming to take me away from here. I want my mother." Pt. is 90 years old.)
2. To illustrate **denial.** (*Example:* Pt. insists, "I don't need any help at home. I'll be fine once I get home." Pt. is dependent for transfers and ambulation and lives alone.)
3. To illustrate a patient's **attitude toward therapy.** (*Example:* Pt. states, "I don't want to play children's games. If I could just go home, I would be fine.")
4. To illustrate the patient's **use of abusive language.** (*Example:* Pt. yelled to therapist, "Keep your hands off my arm! I'm going to kill you!")

> **c/o:** Pt. c/o pain R shoulder when R arm is hanging down and when attempting to put on sweater and T-shirts. **Hx:** States his shoulder started to ache for no apparent reason. Denies having previous injury or trauma to shoulder. **Home situation:** States lives alone. Has only a few clothing items he can get into without help. **Environment/pt.'s goals:** States he has been practicing volleyball 6 hr/day for the last 3 weeks. Wants to play on the college volleyball team this winter.

FIGURE 5–4 The documentation in Figure 5–3 rewritten with the information grouped according to topics.

1) Patient states she's allergic to perfume; itched at treatment site following yesterday's treatment. 2) Patient states he is anxious to go fishing; has six steps down to the dock at his cabin. 3) Patient reports he awoke only three times last night; denies having leg tingling and back soreness.

FIGURE 5–5   Documentation using the word "patient" once.

1. Patient rates pain a 6 on an ascending scale of 1–10 when climbing stairs.
2. Patient gives her pain a 4 on a pain scale of 1–7 where 1 is no pain and 7 is excruciating pain.
3. Patient reports his pain is 3/10 after massage compared to 6/10 before massage.
4. 1_____x_____1
   1 2 3 4 5 6 7 8 9 10

FIGURE 5–6   How documentation of pain looks like objective data.

There are many words that describe pain. Some of these are grouped below. Check (✔) any words that describe the pain you have these days.

1.	5.	9.	13.	17.
Flickering	Pinching	Dull	Fearful	Spreading
Quivering	Pressing	Sore	Frightful	Radiating
Pulsing	Gnawing	Hurting	Terrifying	Penetrating
Throbbing	Cramping	Aching		Piercing
Beating	Crushing	Heavy		
Pounding				
2.	**6.**	**10.**	**14.**	**18.**
Jumping	Tugging	Tender	Punishing	Tight
Flashing	Pulling	Taut	Grueling	Numb
Shooting	Wrenching	Rasping	Cruel	Drawing
		Splitting	Vicious	Squeezing
			Killing	Tearing
3.	**7.**	**11.**	**15.**	**19.**
Pricking	Hot	Tiring	Wretched	Cool
Boring	Burning	Exhausting	Blinding	Cold
Drilling	Scalding			Freezing
Stabbing	Searing			
4.	**8.**	**12.**	**16.**	**20.**
Sharp	Tingling	Sickening	Annoying	Nagging
Cutting	Itchy	Suffocating	Troublesome	Nauseating
Lacerating	Smarting		Miserable	Agonizing
	Stinging		Intense	Dreadful
			Unbearable	Torturing

FIGURE 5–7   An example of a description checklist pain profile. (Adapted from the McGill Pain Questionnaire.)

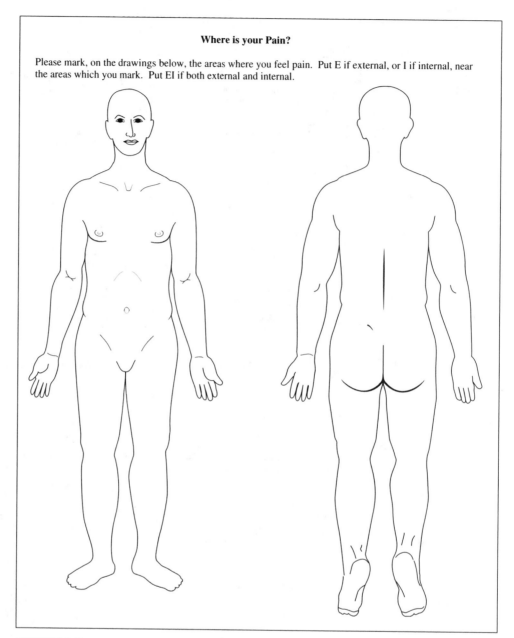

FIGURE 5–8 An example of a body drawing pain profile.

Information Taken from Someone Other Than the Patient

Relevant information is often provided by the caretaker or significant other. This is especially true for patients with dementia, speech dysfunction, infants, young children, and patients who are in a coma.

When the information is provided by someone other than the patient, begin the subjective information by stating who provided the information, and state the reason why the patient could not communicate. (*Example:* All of the following information is provided by pt.'s mother. Pt. is in a coma.)

When information is provided by both the patient and another person, it should be noted when it is patient-supplied information and when the information is supplied by the other person. (*Example:* Mrs. Jones states she did not have to help her husband button his sweater today. Mr. Jones states that today is the first time he has not had to ask for help since his arthritis flared up.)

A Special Word
About Pain

Pain is an element of the subjective data content. Pain information is placed in the S (subjective) section of the SOAP-organized progress note. Documentation of pain is unique because it often seems like objective data (Fig. 5–6) or it may seem as though the presence of pain is the judgment or opinion of the therapist.

The patient is experiencing the pain, and the perception of the intensity of the pain varies among individuals. We have all compared dental experiences with friends. Some never need local anesthesia to have a cavity filled, whereas others need Novocain, music in headphones, and other distractions. Pain is difficult to describe in words, and descriptions are interpreted differently by each person. Since the patient is providing the pain description, this information is documented in the subjective section.

DOCUMENTING PAIN   Each facility has its own procedure for documenting pain. Typically this information is documented in the pain profile. Several types of pain profiles are commonly used:

> **Pain Scale:** Frequently facilities use a pain profile based on a numbered scale, usually from 0–10 or 1–7. The patient rates the pain on the scale, and this is recorded in the subjective section (see Fig. 5–6). The scale should be described in the note (e.g., "0 = no pain, 10 = worst pain imaginable"; "1 = no pain, 7 = excruciating"; "on an ascending scale of 0–10.")
>
> **Checklist of Descriptions:** Another method of documenting pain is a checklist of words describing pain. The patient checks the words that describe his pain. This checklist is inserted in the medical chart, and a note in the subjective section of the progress note instructs the reader to refer to the checklist. Figure 5–7 is an example of a description checklist pain profile.
>
> **Body Drawing:** An outline drawing of the body may be used for the patient to mark the location of the pain on the drawing. Symbols or colors are used to indicate the type and/or intensity of the pain at each location. This is then inserted in the medical chart for pain documentation. Figure 5–8 is an example of a body drawing pain profile.

The pain profile or technique for documenting the pain *must* be consistent in each note. Changes in the pain profile can be identified by a comparison of the pain reports throughout the treatment sessions with the initial profile. Inconsistent documentation hinders a determination of treatment effectiveness. Information on a pain scale cannot be compared with information on a body drawing. Consistent pain documentation provides a clear picture or measurement of treatment effectiveness and helps to ensure reimbursement by third-party payers. It is important to understand that pain profiles provide an objective method for documenting pain, but the profile is documented in the *subjective* section of the progress note. Students often make the mistake of documenting pain in the objective section.

SUMMARY

Information that is told to the PT or PTA by the patient, significant other, or another caregiver is documented as subjective data in the progress note. The information must be relevant to the patient's treatment and/or physical therapy problem. Suggestions about listening for and identifying relevant information are presented. The information can be paraphrased or quoted verbatim. Comments regarding pain and structured pain profiles are documented with the subjective data. It is not necessary to include subjective information in the progress note when none was provided or when the patient repeated information that had already been documented in previous notes.

REVIEW EXERCISES

1. Define subjective data.

2. Discuss the type of subjective data that is relevant to the patient and that should be included in the progress note.

3. Describe the organization of the subjective data.

4. Explain guidelines for writing the subjective data content.

5. Explain why information about pain is subjective data.

6. Describe two mistakes students often make when writing subjective data.

IDENTIFYING THE PHYSICAL THERAPY PROBLEM AND SUBJECTIVE DATA STATEMENTS

Write "Pr" next to statements that describe the physical therapy problem and "SD" next to statements that fit the subjective data category.

_____ Pt. states she has a clear understanding of her disease and her prognosis.

_____ Pt. expresses surprise that the ice massage relaxed her muscle spasm.

_____ Muscle spasms L lumbar paraspinals with sitting tolerance limited to 10 min.

_____ Pt. describes tingling pain down back of R leg to heel.

_____ Dependent in ADLs due to flaccid paralysis in R upper and lower extremities.

_____ Sue states her L ear hurts.

_____ Unable to reach behind back due to limited ROM in R shoulder int. rot.

_____ Reports he must be able to return to work as a welder.

_____ Laceration of R vastus medialis.

_____ Paraplegic 2° SCI T12 and dependent in wheelchair transfers.

_____ States Hx of RA since 1980.

_____ Pt. denies pain c̄ cough.

_____ States injury occurred December 31, 1994.

_____ SPTA c/o he has to sit for 2 hours in the PTA lectures.

_____ Grip strength weakness and inability to turn doorknobs to open doors due to carpal tunnel syndrome.

_____ Describes his pain as "burning."

_____ Unable to sit due to decubitus over sacrum.

_____ Unable to feed self due to limited elbow flexion.

_____ Pt. rates her pain a 4 on an ascending scale of 1–10.

_____ States able to sit through a 2-hour movie last night.

1. Identify the statements in Practice Exercise 1 to which you answered "Pr." *Underline* the neuromusculoskeletal problem (impairment) and *circle* the functional limitation.

2. *Underline* the verb in the statements that clued you to identify the statements as "SD."

3. List the medical diagnosis you can find in the statements.

_____

_____

_____

_____

_____

You are treating Nancy who has been diagnosed as having a mild disc protrusion at L4,5 with spasms in the right lumbar paraspinal muscles. You read in the PT initial evaluation that she reported pain in right low back and buttock areas, and you see the areas marked on a body drawing. The spasms and pain have caused Nancy to be unable to tolerate sitting longer than 15 minutes and unable to sleep more than 2 hours at a time, and she reports having difficulty with bathing and dressing activities. Nancy works as a nursing assistant at the local hospital and has been unable to perform her job tasks. The desired functional outcomes are for Nancy to be able to sit 30 minutes, sleep 5 hours, achieve independence in bathing and dressing, and return to her work as a nursing assistant. The treatment plan and objectives are massage to the lumbar paraspinal muscles to relax the spasms, 10 minutes of static pelvic traction to encourage the disc protrusion to recede and to stretch and relax the lumbar paraspinal muscles, patient education in a home exercise program for lumbar extension and control of the disc protrusion, and posture and body mechanics instructions for correct and safe sitting, sleeping, bathing, dressing, and performance of work tasks. You have written this progress note:

6-3-94:   **Dx:** Disc protrusion L4,5.

Pr: Muscle spasms lumbar paraspinals with limited sitting, sleeping tolerance, difficulty with ADLs, and unable to perform work tasks.

Patient states she was able to sit through 30 minutes of *The Young and The Restless* soap opera yesterday. Rates her pain a 5 on an ascending scale of 1–10. Patient has received 4 treatment sessions. Decrease in muscle tone palpable after 10-minute massage to right lumbar paraspinal muscles, prone position over one thin pillow. Unable to tolerate lying propped on elbows due to pain before traction, able to lie propped on elbows 5 minutes following 10 minutes, prone, static pelvic traction, 70 pounds. No pain in buttock area. Correctly performed lumbar extension exercises 1, 2, and 3 of home exercise program (see copy in chart) and observed consistently using correct sitting posture with lumbar roll. Patient required frequent verbal cuing for correct body mechanics while performing 10 repetitions (3 reps in initial eval.) of circuit of job simulation activities consisting of bed making, rolling, and moving 30-pound (10-pound in initial eval.) dummy "patient" in bed, pivot transferring the dummy, and wheelchair handling. She did 10 back arches between each task without reminders. Patient has reached 30-minute sitting tolerance goal, is independent with home exercise program and compliant with techniques for controlling the protrusion. Progress toward outcome of return to work is 60% with more consistent use of correct body mechanics and ability to lift 50-pound dummy required. Patient to continue treatment sessions 3×/week for 2 more weeks per PT's initial plan. Will notify PT that interim evaluation is scheduled for 6-7-94.

Sue Smith, PTA, Lic. #0003

Describe what you have done wrong in writing this note and rewrite it correctly.

Place "Yes" next to relevant subjective data statements and "No" next to those that do not seem relevant.

_____ Client stated her dog was hit by a car last night and she felt too depressed today to do her exercises.

_____ Client reported he progressed his exercises to 50 push-ups yesterday.

_____ Patient's daughter stated she traveled from Iowa, where it has been raining for 2 weeks.

_____ Patient states he does not like the hospital food and is hungry for some Dairy Queen.

_____ Patient rates her pain a 4 on an ascending scale of 1–7.

_____ Patient states she is now able to reach the second shelf of her kitchen cupboard to reach for a glass.

_____ Patient reports he had this same tingling discomfort in his right foot 3 years ago.

_____ Client reports experiencing an aching in his "elbow bone" after the ultrasound treatment yesterday.

_____ Patient says she has 10 grandchildren and 4 great grandchildren.

_____ Client states she forgot to tell the PT that she loves to bowl.

_____ Client reports that *Northern Exposure* is his favorite TV program.

_____ Client reports he sat in his fishing boat 3 hours and caught a 7-pound Northern this weekend.

_____ Client states he played golf yesterday for the first time since his back injury.

_____ Client states he shot a 56 in golf.

_____ Client states she cannot turn her head to look over her shoulder to back the car out of the garage.

_____ Patient's mother wants to know when her son will come out of the coma.

_____ Client reports he wishes he had not been drinking beer the night of his accident.

_____ Patient describes his flight of stairs with 10 steps, a landing, then 5 more steps and the railing on the right when going up.

_____ Client wishes it would rain, as her prize roses are dying.

_____ Patient states, "I'm going to Macy's to shop and have lunch today." (Patient is 89 years old and is a resident in a long-term care facility in a small town in Ohio. She has been placed on some new medication.)

Writing the Content: Objective Data

Learning Objectives

After studying this chapter, the student will be able to:

- Recognize objective data information
- Organize objective data information for easy reading and understanding
- Follow recommended guidelines for documenting objective data information
- Document the patient's functional abilities so the reader can picture the patient functioning
- Document treatment so that it is reproducible by another PTA or a PT
- Document objective data consistent with the data in the PT's initial evaluation
- Identify common mistakes students typically make when documenting objective data

The **objective data** in the PT's evaluation and the PTA's progress note are included with or immediately after the subjective data. These data make up the content of the O (objective) section of the SOAP outline and are included in the content of the data section of the DEP note. This information is part of the status information in the PSPG-organized note and is the physical therapy assessment information in the FOR.

The reader of the objective data in the PTA's progress note should be able to form a mental picture of the patient receiving the treatment, the patient's response to the treatment, and the patient's functioning before and after the treatment. The PTA should write the objective data so that the words paint a picture of the patient and the treatment session.

DEFINITION OF OBJECTIVE DATA

Objective data include any information that can be reproduced or observed by someone else with the same training (i.e., another PT or PTA). It should also be written so that a reader who is not trained in physical therapy can understand the treatment session and determine whether or not the patient is benefiting from physical therapy. The PTA should write the objective section with two audiences in mind: (1) another PTA (imagine you don't feel well, you probably will not come to work tomorrow, and someone else will have to treat your patient); and (2) a reader untrained in physical therapy (e.g., an insurance representative, a lawyer, a quality assurance committee member, a physician, or another health care provider) who is determining the effectiveness of the treatment session.

ORGANIZING AND WRITING THE OBJECTIVE DATA

Five general topics appropriate for the objective data in the progress note are (1) results of measurements and/or tests, (2) description of the patient's function, (3) description of the treatment provided, (4) objective observations of the patient made by the PTA, and (5) record of treatment sessions.

Organizing the Objective Data

The information in the objective section of the progress note should be organized so that it flows from one topic to the next and is easy to read. The PTA should group similar information together: For example, treatment descriptions, results of measurements and/or tests, and descriptions of the patient's functioning should be organized into three distinct groups.

Writing the Objective Data

The objective data in the initial evaluation must consist of information that is relevant to the patient's chief complaint and the reason the patient is seeking physical therapy care. These data form the basis for designing the treatment goals and plan. The objective data should be written in measurable terms so that the efficacy of physical therapy treatment procedures can be determined through research of the progress note. When appropriate, the PTA should relate the progress note objective data information to the same information in the initial evaluation and/or previous notes for comparison. Some objective data can be charted or graphed for a quick picture of progress.

The Results of Measurements and/or Tests

Activities or areas specifically mentioned in the initial evaluation and goals should be reassessed and recorded in the progress notes and in the interim and discharge evaluations. The PTA assesses the patient's progress by readministering the measurements and/or tests performed in the initial evaluation that the PTA is trained to perform. A comparison is made with the results in either the initial evaluation or in previous progress notes if the patient has been receiving physical therapy for a long period of time. For the comparison to be valid, the retest or measurement must follow the same procedures and techniques as were performed in the initial evaluation. The documentation of the results must also be consistent. For example, if the measurements were in centimeters in the initial evaluation, they should continue to be documented in centimeters.

The documentation of the results may be in the form of either a comment referring the reader to previous results (e.g., "See distance walked in note dated 8-2-93") or an actual written comparison with the results of the previous measurements or tests.

Example: PTA Sam is treating Mr. Wilson with compression pump to decrease edema in the L ankle. Measurements of the circumference of Mr. Wilson's L ankle were taken in the initial evaluation (on 8-10-94) to determine the extent of the edema. Today, after 5 treatments, Sam remeasures the circumference of the ankle and compares his results with the initial evaluation measurements to prove that the edema has decreased and the compression pump treatments are effective.

Sam could record the measurements in a chart form in the objective section for easy comparison. Figure 6–1 illustrates the measurement results in a chart form.

It is easy for the reader to compare results and see that the edema has decreased and the patient is benefiting from the compression pump treatment. Another PTA could follow the directions and duplicate the measurement procedure. Other measurements and tests performed by PTAs, with guidelines for documenting the results, are in Figure 6–2.

A Description of the Patient's Function

The PTA documents improvement by describing the patient's **function**.

	8-10-94	8-15-94
Center L lat. malleolus	6"	4"
1" inferior to center L lat. malleolus	5.5"	3"
1" superior to center L lat. malleolus	6"	4"
All measurements taken along the superior edge of the marks.		

FIGURE 6–1 Measurement results in a chart form.

Example: At initial evaluation, Mr. Wilson could not fit his L foot into his running shoe because of the edema in the L foot and ankle. Today, he was able to get his L foot into the shoe with the help of a shoe horn.

The next day another PTA could duplicate the assessment by watching Mr. Wilson use a shoe horn to put on his left running shoe. This is a good way to document treatment effectiveness because it paints a picture of the patient and describes clearly how the physical therapy treatment is improving the patient's ability to function in his environment. The functional activities must be those specifically mentioned in the goals or functional outcomes in the initial evaluation.

When a comparison of the assessment results shows that the patient's functional status has not changed, be sure all methods for measuring change have been used. For example, a patient may continue to need the assistance of one person for ambulation, but the time it takes the patient to walk from bed to bathroom has decreased. The following are suggestions for information to include when describing the patient's function:

Guidelines:
All measurements and tests must be performed and documented in the same manner as they were performed and documented in the PT initial evaluation. The documentation should include, when applicable:
1. Exactly what is being measured or tested, and which side.
2. If it is a motion, is it passive or active?
3. The position of the patient.
4. The starting and ending points, the boundaries, and the measurement points above and below the starting point.
5. The same scale (e.g., inches, centimeters, degrees) that was used in the initial evaluation.

Measurements:
Using the tape measure:
    Girth or circumference
    Leg length
    Wound size
    Step and stride lengths
    Neck and trunk range of motion
Goniometry of all joints

Tests:
Manual muscle test muscle groups
Gross sensory testing

Vital Signs:
Heart rate
Respiratory rate
Blood pressure

Standardized Functional Tests:
These are examples of many tests available:
    Functional Independence Measure (FIM)
    Barthel Assessment
    Tinetti Balance
    Peabody Developmental Motor Scales
    Duke Mobility Skills
    Posture

FIGURE 6–2 Other measurements and tests performed by PTAs, with guidelines for documenting the results.

1. The function (e.g., ambulation, transferring, stair climbing, lifting, sweeping, sitting, standing, moving from sit to stand or stand to sit)
2. Description of the quality of the movement when performing the function (e.g., even weight bearing, smooth movement, correct body mechanics, speed)
3. Level of assistance needed (i.e., ranging from independent to verbal reminders; tactile guidance; supervision; standby assist or contact guard, minimal, moderate, maximal; to dependent)
4. Purpose of the assistance (e.g., verbal cuing for gait pattern, for recovery of loss of balance, for added strength, to monitor weight bearing, to guide walker)
5. Description of equipment needed (e.g., ambulation aids, orthotics, supports, railings, wheelchair, assistive devices)
6. Distances, heights, lengths, times, weights (e.g., 300 ft, 10 meters, 6 min, top shelf of standard-height kitchen cabinet, floor to table, 20 lb)
7. Environmental conditions (e.g., level surface, carpeting, dim light, outside, ramps, low seat)

STANDARDIZED FUNCTIONAL ASSESSMENTS For assessing functional abilities, there are many tools that have set protocols and procedures, clear instructions, and a method for rating or scoring the level of function. Examples of these tests are the Tinetti Balance Test, the Peabody Developmental Motor Scales, the Barthel Assessment, Duke Mobility Skills, and Functional Independence Measure. If a standardized assessment tool is used in the initial evaluation, the PTA, when trained in the use of the tool, can reassess the patient's functional abilities and refer the reader of the progress note to the copy of the completed assessment form in the chart. The assessment tool describes the function and changes in the rating score as evidence of improvement in functional abilities.

A Description of the Treatment Provided

The objective data may include information about the treatment the patient received. Facilities differ as to how treatment details are recorded. The treatment may be described in the progress note, recorded on a flow chart, or described on a separate form elsewhere in the chart, or it may be a combination of narrative progress notes with a check-off chart. Besides being recorded in the medical record, the treatment is often detailed on a cardex located in the physical therapy department. The PTA should follow the procedures of the facility.

Treatment details must be complete enough so that the treatment can be duplicated by another PT or PTA. The following information should be included for the treatment description to be reproducible.

1. Identification of the modality, exercise, or activity
2. Dosage, number of repetitions, and distance
3. Identification of the exact piece of equipment, when applicable
4. Settings of dials or programs on equipment
5. Target tissue or treatment area
6. Purpose of the treatment
7. Patient positioning
8. Duration, frequency, and rest breaks
9. Anything the therapist needs to do or be aware of that is outside standard procedure or protocol
10. Anything that is unique to the treatment of that particular patient

Appendix B provides guidelines for documentation of specific modalities and treatment procedures.

The treatment description should include or be combined with a description of the patient's **response** to the treatment.

Example: Decreased muscle spasm (decreased tone) was palpable following ice massage, to numbing response (7 min), L paraspinal mms, L3–5, with pt. prone over one pillow.

The treatment details can be included to describe **function.**

O: Following verbal instructions and demonstrations, pt. accurately performed home exercise program designed to strengthen R hip abductors, extensors, and quadriceps, 5 reps of each ex. today. Pt. provided written instructions, refer to copy in chart.

O: Pt. accurately demonstrated set-up of home cervical polyaxial traction unit; gave self 10-min intermittent traction,15 lb, approximately 5 sec on, 3 sec off, supine. Pt. provided written instructions, see copy in chart.

FIGURE 6–3 Objective documentation of a treatment session that included instructing the patient in a home exercise program.

Example: Following instructions, pt. safely ambulated with axillary crutches, no wt. bearing on L, from bed to dining room (50 ft) on tiled level surface with standby assist for support for loss of balance recovery 2×.

In these two examples, a reader who is untrained in physical therapy can visualize the patient's performance, and another PTA could duplicate the treatment the following day.

A copy of any written instructions or information provided to the patient as part of the treatment should be placed in the medical record. Frequently the PTA will give the patient and/or a caregiver written instructions for exercises or activities that were taught during the treatment session. This is noted in the objective data, and the reader is informed that a copy is in the chart. When the reader can reproduce the treatment by following the written instructions on the handout, it is not necessary to describe the exercises in the progress note. Figure 6–3 illustrates objective documentation of a treatment session that includes instructing the patient in a home exercise program. In the objective data section, any equipment that was given, loaned, or sold to the patient should be mentioned.

The PTA's Objective Observations of the Patient

A description of what the PTA sees or feels (visual and tactile observations) constitutes objective data if it is an observation that another PT or PTA would also make because they have the same training. The observation could be duplicated or confirmed by another PT or PTA. Two examples of objective observations are (1) reddened skin over a bony area after application of hot packs and (2) a description of the patient's gait pattern or how the patient walks.

11-12-93: Pr: Sciatic nerve pain limiting sitting tolerance due to disc protrusion L4–5.

S: Pt. stated he has pain extending down back of R leg, and it came on "all of a sudden" while moving his TV set. He wished he could sit long enough to watch his son's hockey games. After traction and treatment, pt. reported pain no longer in leg but located in low back.

O: Pt. demonstrated frequent wt. shifting and position changing while sitting for 15 min prior to tx. Gave mech. static lumbar traction to L4–5 area, 10 min, 90 lb, pt. prone over 1 pillow, table split, to decrease protrusion and pressure on nerve to decrease pain. Instructed pt. in ADL body mechanics, how to maintain lumbar lordosis at all times, and explained the process of a protruded disc. Instructed how to get on/off bed. Gave home instructions of McKenzie extension exercises.

A: _____

P: _____

_____ Steven Student, SPTA/Mary Smith, PT Lic #4321

5-3-93: Pr: Flexed posture, shuffling gait due to Parkinson's disease.

S: Pt. states his legs feel stiff and he stumbles frequently. Feels he needs to hold on to something when he walks.

O: Pt. observed using shuffling gait with hips, knees, and trunk in slight flexion. Min. knee flexion during pre-swing and initial swing. Instructed pt. how to walk with front-wheeled rolling walker, instructed heel to toe. Did reciprocal inhibition to quads to relax quads and increase knee flexion.

A: _____

P: _____

_____ Susan Student, SPTA/Paul Jones, PTA Lic #007

FIGURE 6–4 Examples of students' common mistake of writing the objective section of the progress note in terms of what they did.

11-12-93: **Pr:** Sciatic nerve pain limiting sitting tolerance due to disc protrusion L4–5.

S: Pt. states he has pain extending down back of R leg, and it came on "all of a sudden" while moving his TV set. He wishes he could sit long enough to watch his son's hockey games. After traction & treatment, pt. reports pain no longer in leg but is located in low back.

O: Pt. demonstrated frequent wt. shifting and position changing while sitting for 15 min prior to tx. tx: mech. static lumbar traction to L4–5 area, 10 min, 90 lb, prone over 1 pillow, table split, to decrease protrusion and pressure on nerve to decrease pain. Pt. demonstrated an understanding of spine and disc anatomy education, as well as instructions in maintaining a lumbar lordosis and correct body mechanics for ADLs by giving correct return demonstrations of lifting/reaching/bending/pushing/pulling body mechanics, by maintaining his lumbar lordosis when getting up off of the traction table, and by sitting without wt. shifts for 15 min using lumbar cushion. Pt. correctly performed McKenzie extension exercises per written instructions (see copy in chart).

A: _____

P: _____

_____ Steven Student, SPA/Mary Smith, PT Lic. #4321

5-3-93: **Pr:** Flexed posture, shuffling gait due to Parkinson's disease.

S: Pt. states his legs feel stiff and he stumbles frequently. Feels he needs to hold on to something when he walks.

O: Pt. observed using shuffling gait with hips, and trunk in slight flexion. Min. knee flexion during pre-swing and initial swing. After 3 reps, reciprocal inhibition exercise to quads bil, sitting, to relax the muscles and encourage knee flexion; pt. demonstrated improved knee flexion during the swing phase of gait. Pt. ambulated with a front-wheeled rolling walker, 100 ft in PT depart. on tiled floor, 3X with SBA for frequent verbal cues for heel–toe gait pattern and knee flexion. Pt. demonstrated erect posture with walker.

A: _____

P: _____

_____ Susan Student, SPTA/Paul Jones, PTA Lic. #007

FIGURE 6–5   The notes in Figure 4–4 written correctly, in terms of what the *patient* did.

Example 1: A nickel-size, reddened area noted over inferior angle of left scapular after hot pack treatment.

Example 2: Client walks with an antalgic gait; trunk held in a slightly forward-leaning posture, minimal arm swing, no pelvic rotation, uneven step length (shorter on right), and shortened stance time on right.

Record of Treatment Sessions   When a third-party payer has limited the number of treatment sessions provided a patient, the progress note can be a method for tracking the number of sessions. The objective data section can contain a report as to the number of times the patient has been treated, and the information in the plan section of the note can state how many more treatment sessions are scheduled in the future.

5-3-93: **Pr:** No knee extension during gait due to biceps femoris tendon tear.

S: Pt. states she feels more comfortable walking after US tx.

O: Direct contact US/1 MHz/0.7 w/cm^2/5 min/CW/mild heat, prone to biceps femoris insertion to increase circulation, and promote healing of tendon. Working on increasing R knee extension for initial contact. Quadriceps, hip flexors F+ strength (F in initial eval.). R knee AROM before tx, 20–100°, after tx 15–100°. Manual resistance strengthening exercise to quadriceps and hip flexors with isometric contractions at end of range, 10X each, 6-sec hold. Instructed in home exercises (see chart). Assessed FWB gait, no R heel contact. Pt. correctly demonstrated home exercises.

A: _____

P: _____

_____ Jim Citizen, SPTA/Tom Jones, PT Lic #1006

FIGURE 6–6   A disorganized objective section of the progress note in which the information rambles.

5-3-93: **Pr:** No knee extension during gait due to right biceps femoris tendon tear.
   S: Pt. states she feels more comfortable walking after US tx.
   O: Pt. demonstrated FWB gait but does not fully extend right knee at initial contact. After US and exercise treatment, pt. was able consciously to improve knee extension at initial contact. Direct contact US/1MHz/0.7w/cm²/CW/mild heat, prone to right biceps femoris insertion to increase circulation, promote healing of tendon, and gain knee extension for initial contact in gait. Right quadriceps, hip flexors F+ strength (F in initial eval). Manual resistance strengthening exercise to right quads and hip flexors with isometric contractions at end of range, sitting, 10X each, 6- sec hold. Pt. correctly demonstrated home exercises to strengthen quads and hip flexors and gentle stretching exercises for hamstrings to gain knee extension during gait (see copy of written instructions in chart). R knee AROM before tx 20–100°, after tx 15-100°.
   A: _____
   P: _____
   _____ Jim Citizen, SPTA/Tom Jones, PT Lic #1006

FIGURE 6–7 The note in Figure 6–6 rewritten with the information organized.

Common Mistakes Students Make When Documenting the Objective Data

The major mistake PTA students make when writing objective data, especially when documenting the treatment provided, is reporting what *they* did and not how the *patient* responded or performed, (e.g., "Instructed pt. in crutch walking, non–wt. bearing L). This statement refers to what the therapist did and does not give the reader a picture of the patient's performance. The progress note is about *the patient* and should be written so that it describes the patient's response to the treatment plan and progress toward the goals. Examples of progress notes written by students describing what they did are in Figure 6–4. Figure 6–5 illustrates those notes rewritten in terms of the patient's response.

The tendency to ramble is another common problem students have when first learning to document. Organizing the information according to topics prevents rambling. Figure 6–6 is an example of an unorganized objective section of a progress note. Figure 6–7 is the same note, but with the information grouped by topic.

SUMMARY

The objective data content of the progress note provides proof that the treatment was given, information as to the effectiveness of the treatment, and evidence as to whether or not the patient is improving. This content must be measurable and reproducible. This may include treatment details, a comparison of results of measurements and/or tests with previous results, visual and tactile observations made by the PTA, and descriptions of the patient's functional abilities. It should be written so that the words paint a picture of the patient and the treatment session and so that the reader can visualize how the patient is functioning. The objective data content must be relevant to the chief complaint, the goals or functional outcomes, and the reason for the physical therapy treatment.

REVIEW EXERCISES

1. Describe the criteria for information to be considered objective data.

2. List the types of information included in the objective data content.

3. Describe how results of test and measurements are documented.

4. Explain what information should be included when describing the patient's function.

5. Describe what information should be included for the treatment to be reproducible.

6. Describe mistakes students commonly make when documenting objective data.

IDENTIFYING THE PROBLEM, SUBJECTIVE DATA, AND OBJECTIVE DATA STATEMENTS

Write "Pr" next to the problem statements, "SD" next to the subjective data statements, and "OD" next to the objective data statements.

_____ Pt. c/o pain with prolonged sitting.

_____ Decubitus on sacrum measures 3 cm from L outer edge to R outer edge.

_____ Pt. ambulates with ataxic gait, 10 ft max. assist of 2 to prevent fall.

_____ R knee flexion PROM 30–90°.

_____ Ambulates c̄ standard walker, PWB L, bed to bathroom (20 ft), tiled surface, min. assist 1× for balance, verbal cuing for gait pattern.

_____ Pt. states he is fearful of crutch walking.

_____ Limited ROM in L shoulder 2° to Fx greater tubercle of humerus and unable to put on winter coat without help.

_____ c/o itching in scar R knee.

_____ Transfers: supine ↔ sit c̄ min. assist 1× for strength.

_____ Unable to feed self with L hand because of limited elbow ROM 2° Fx L olecranon process.

_____ AROM WNL bil. LEs.

_____ Pt. demonstrated adequate knee flexion during initial swing c̄ verbal cuing p̄ hamstring exercises.

_____ Dependent in bed mobility due to dislocated R hip.

_____ Expresses concern over lack of progress.

_____ L shoulder flexion PROM 0–100°, lat. rot. PROM 0–40°.

_____ Kathy reports PTA courses are easy.

_____ Pt. pivot transfers, NWB R, bed ↔ w/c, max assist 2× for strength, balance, NWB cuing.

_____ Pt. rates L knee pain 5/10 when going up stairs.

_____ LUE circumference at 3 cm superior to olecranon process is 12 cm.

_____ BP 125/80 mmHg, pulse 78 BPM, regular, strong.

Use the list of statements in Practice Exercise 1 as well as your answers to them.
1. In the "Pr" statements, *underline* the musculoskeletal problem and *circle* the functional limitation.
2. In the "SD" statements, underline the key *verb* that led you to write "SD."
3. In the "OD" statements, underline the key *information* that led you to write "OD."
4. List the medical diagnoses you can find in the statements.

_____

_____

_____

_____

_____

Refer to the general documentation guidelines in Figure 6–2, and critique each of the following statements that document the results of a test or measurement. Write what is missing or wrong, if anything, in the documentation.

1. Left knee flexion PROM 0–63° in sitting position (0–55° in initial eval.).

_____

_____

2. Decubitus over sacrum 3.25 inches from left border to right border, 7 cm in initial eval.

_____

_____

3. Hip ROM 75°.

_____

_____

_____

4. Hip abductor strength G−, 3/5 in initial eval.

_____

_____

5. Left hip hyperextension with anterior pelvic tilt, prone, 20°.

_____

_____

6. Circumference at right olecranon process 4 inches, upper arm 6 inches, lower arm 3 inches.

_____

_____

7. Blood pressure 120/70, pulse 72.

_____

_____

8. Circumference right wrist, supine, UE elevated 45°, 3rd metacarpal head 8 inches, 2 inches superior to 3rd metacarpal head 8 inches, superior edge of ulnar styloid process 7 cm, taken along superior border of marks.

_____

_____

9. Resting respiratory rate 12 breaths per minute relaxed, quiet, sitting position.

_____

_____

10. Left shoulder flexion 100°, abduction 100°, external rotation 60°, internal rotation 40°.

_____

_____

11. Left knee flexion PROM, prone with towel under thigh, 20–110° (30–90° initial eval.).

_____

_____

12. Right leg 1 inch longer than left.

_____

_____

13. Trunk forward bend 20%.

_____

_____

14. Trunk side bend greater on right than left.

_____

_____

15. Cervical rotation to right 0–25°, aligned with nose, sitting position, shoulders stabilized.

_____

_____

PRACTICE EXERCISE 4

Refer to documentation guidelines in Figure 6–2 and suggestions for documenting modalities in Appendix B, and then critique the following statements documenting modality treatment. Could you reproduce the treatment? If not, what is missing?

1. US/1.5 w/cm^2/right shoulder.

_____

_____

2. Low back massage.

_____

_____

_____

_____

3. Strengthening exercises consisting of quad. sets, hamstring sets, and glut. sets/right/5 sec hold/10 reps each/supine/following 1 hr on knee CPM.

_____

_____

4. Exercises to increase ROM left shoulder.

_____

_____

5. Cervical traction/15 min/14 lb/to stretch muscles.

_____

_____

6. Tilt table/20 min/45°.

_____

_____

7. Home exercise program to increase left knee ROM and strengthen left quadriceps for stair climbing to get to upstairs bathroom (see copy in chart).

_____

_____

8. Phonophoresis/left/subacromial bursa/sitting/to decrease inflammation.

_____

_____

9. High voltage E-stim/motor response/right rhomboids & middle trapezius/to relax spasms.

_____

_____

10. Mechanical pelvic traction/intermittent/30 sec on, 10 sec off/supine (90–90)/90 lb/30 min/to encourage posterior pelvic tilt and stretch lumbar extensor muscles/to decrease lordotic posture.

_____

_____

The following are treatment scenarios in which you are the PTA working on functional activities with your patients. *Paint a picture* of each patient's functioning as if being recorded in the objective data section of your progress note. It is not difficult to paint a picture of the patient's functioning. Just mentally reproduce the treatment session and write the description of the patient performing the activity and how the patient responded to what you are doing. Refer to page 80 for documentation guidelines.

1. You instructed Mrs. Smith, who has severely sprained her right ankle, in crutch walking using a non–weight-bearing gait. Her ankle has been casted, and she is not allowed to bear weight on the right for 3 days. You fitted her with axillary crutches and taught her how to walk 100 ft on tiled and carpeted level surfaces; how to sit down and get up from bed, chair, and toilet; how to climb a flight of stairs with the railing on the right going up; how to manage curbs and two steps without using a railing; and how to get in and out of her car. Mrs. Smith safely ambulated and required only verbal cuing from you to climb the stairs. You gave her written crutch-walking instructions.

_____

_____

_____

_____

_____

_____

_____

2. You supervised Jack practicing his circuit of job-simulation activities using correct body mechanics for 20 minutes, 15 repetitions. Jack has had back surgery (laminectomy L4,5) and is preparing to return to work as a bricklayer. You observed that he consistently maintained his correct lumbar curve when squatting to lift bricks and weight shifting to spread the mortar. He did need body mechanics reminders when he lifted the wheelbarrow handles and while wheeling the wheelbarrow, especially for turns. He tended to bend from the waist to reach the handles and to twist his trunk when turning the wheelbarrow.

_____

_____

_____

_____

_____

_____

_____

3. You taught Sally, a paraplegic from a spinal cord injury, how to transfer from her wheelchair to the toilet using a sliding board. She required constant instructions and cuing regarding safety precautions, and you needed to help push her across the board. You felt as though you did most of the work. The third time she tried, she was able to slide herself from the chair to the toilet with only a little boost from you. However, when going from the toilet to the chair, it felt as though you and Sally exerted equal effort.

_____

_____

_____

_____

_____

_____

4. You worked with Mr. Olson on ambulation with a wide-base quad cane in his left hand. He had a stroke and has right upper and lower extremity weakness. You walked with him from his bed into the bathroom, to the bedroom window, out into the hall area in front of his door, and back to his wheelchair next to the bed. He walked this circuit five times, with a 2-minute rest in the wheelchair between each trip. You needed to hold his gait belt and to assist him in shifting his weight to his right leg. He stumbled three times, but he was able to recover his balance without your help. During the fourth and fifth trips, he was able to weight shift to the right appropriately without your help.

_____

_____

_____

_____

_____

_____

Writing the Content: Problems, Goals or Functional Outcomes, and Treatment Effectiveness

Learning Objectives

After studying this chapter, the student will be able to:

- Describe the significance of the subjective and objective data in the progress note
- Recognize the qualities of a properly written goal
- Discuss why the interpretation of the data is the most important portion of the progress note
- Explain the topics that should be included when the PTA interprets the progress note data
- Connect the information in the progress note to the information in the PT's initial evaluation
- Write a progress note without making common mistakes

Subjective and objective data are informative facts. After reviewing the data, the reader may ask, "So what?" Providing content consisting of **problems, goals or functional outcomes,** and **treatment effectiveness** answers that question. *This content provides the rationale for the necessity of the physical therapy medical treatment.* The interpretation and significance of the subjective and objective data are reflected in the initial evaluation by the identification of the physical therapy problem and the design of the treatment goals. The PTA documents the significance of the data in the progress note by describing the results of the treatment and the patient's progress toward the accomplishment of the treatment goals. This information is located in the A (assessment) section of the SOAP outline and the E (evaluation) section of the DEP format, and it is the content contained in the problems and functional outcome goals portions of the FOR. The information is scattered throughout the PSPG-organized progress note. The physical therapy problem constitutes the first P (problem) section. The rationale for modified treatment plans contained in the second P (plan) section is based on the significance of the data. Discussion about progress toward goals is provided in the G section. For ease of discussion in this chapter, the information will be referred to as **interpretation of the data content.**

Interpretation of the data content is more complex in the PT's evaluation reports than in the PTA's progress notes.

INTERPRETATION OF THE DATA CONTENT

Interpretation of the Data Content in the Evaluation

The APTA's *Guidelines for Physical Therapy Documentation* states that the evaluation report should include the physical therapy diagnosis or problem and the **long-term goals** (LTGs) and **short-term goals** (STGs) to be accomplished.[1] The PT organizing the evaluation information in SOAP format places this information in the A section. This section contains the PT's interpretation of the signs and symptoms, test results, and observations presented during the evaluation process, as well as a conclusion or judgment about the meaning or relevance of the information. The physical therapy problems are determined on the basis of this *interpretation,* and the long- and short-term goals or desired functional outcomes are established on the basis of the *problems.* Thus, the subjective and objective information is summarized, and the "so what?" question is answered.

Writing the Goals and Functional Outcomes

The PT and the patient (or a representative of the patient) collaborate to establish the goals or functional outcomes for the physical therapy treatment. These goals or outcomes relate to the patient's functional limitations or reason he or she is receiving therapy. The LTGs or functional outcomes are the correction or modification of these limitations at the time the patient is discharged from physical therapy. They are broad statements describing the functional abilities necessary for the patient to no longer require physical therapy at that facility. The accomplishment of the long-term functional outcome will eliminate or decrease the severity of the patient's disability. The short-term goals or outcomes are the functional abilities the patient will need to accomplish in order to reach the LTG. The STGs are the steps to the LTG or the desired functional activity broken down into its tasks. The goal or outcome must be written to include the **action** (i.e., the performance) of a function (e.g., will ambulate), **measurable criteria** that determines the accomplishment of the task (e.g., from bedroom to kitchen), and a **time period** within which it is expected the goal or outcome will be met (e.g., in 1 week). Examples of long- and short-term goals or functional outcomes are given in Figure 7–1. Writing the goals in this manner gives the PTA direction for planning treatment sessions that include activities which enable the patient to progress toward the goal, measuring or assessing the patient's progress, and determining when to recommend termination of treatment.

The PTA does not design the treatment goals or functional outcomes, but the PTA can work with the PT in offering suggestions, notifying the PT when goals are met, and recognizing when the PT needs to modify or change goals.

The PTA knows the patient's evaluation results and refers to the goals listed in the evaluation when writing about the interpretation of the progress note data. This coordination of the evaluation and the progress note provides written proof of the PT–PTA team approach to the patient's care and enables the reader to determine the quality of care being provided.

Interpretation of the Data Content in the Progress Note

Interpretation of the data information is the most important section in the progress note. Most readers of the medical record look for this information first because it is the PTA's **summary** of the progress note data with comments about the relevance and meaning of the information. These comments inform the reader of the **effectiveness of the treatment plan** and the progress the patient may or may not be making toward the goals. Any comment made by the PTA must be supported by the subjective and/or objective information. The comments should be grouped or organized so that the information is easy to follow and understand.

A. Situation: Patient had stroke (CVA) 2 weeks ago and is now home, receiving physical therapy 3 times a week through a home health agency. His wife is the caregiver.
Dx: R CVA.
Pr: L hemiparesis with dependent mobility in all aspects.
LTGs: At anticipated discharge date in 1 month:
  1. Patient will ambulate with an assistive device and minimal assist for balance to the bathroom and to meals in 3 weeks.
  2. Patient will be able to manage two steps with an assistive device and a railing as well as car transfers for next visit to the doctor in 4 weeks.
STGs:
  1. Pt. will consistently move up and down in bed, roll from side to side, and when on L side will reach for telephone and call bell with SBA in 2 weeks.
  2. Pt. will consistently move from supine to sitting on edge of bed and return to supine position with minimal assist to help swing L leg into bed in 1 week.
  3. Pt. will consistently move from sitting to standing and back to sitting from bed, toilet, wheelchair, and standard chair with minimum assist for balance control and even weight-bearing cuing in 2 weeks.
  4. Using a quad cane, pt. will consistently ambulate bed to bathroom, and to meals with moderate assist for balance control and gait posture cuing in 2 weeks.
  5. Pt. will manage two steps using quad cane and railing with moderate assist in 3 weeks.

B. Situation: Patient is 1 week postoperation for total hip replacement and is in a subacute rehabilitation unit. Patient is receiving physical therapy 2X/day with plans to be discharged to home.
Dx: L total hip replacement
Pr: Weakened hip musculature and dependent in rising from sit to stand and ambulation.
LTGs: At anticipated discharge in 20 days, patient will transfer and ambulate independently for return to home.
  1. Patient will independently and consistently move from sit to stand and stand to sit using elevated toilet seat, and all other surfaces no lower than 18 inches.
  2. Patient will independently and consistently walk with a straight cane on all surfaces and in the community.
STGs:
  1. Pt. will consistently be able to sit to stand and return with SBA if boost is needed from edge of bed, elevated toilet seat, wheelchair, and standard dining room chair in 10 days.
  2. Pt. will consistently be able to ambulate using a straight cane for balance on tiled and carpeted level surfaces, to bathroom and dining room for meals with SBA for balance control in 10 days.

FIGURE 7–1   Examples of long-term goals/functional outcomes and short-term goals/outcomes.

Change in the Impairment

A summary of the meaning of results of measurements, tests, or observations recorded in the objective data can describe a change in the impairment severity compared with the status of the patient at the initial evaluation. For example, if the objective data include girth measurements of the patient's arm that are less than the results of previous measurements and the patient's elbow flexion measurements show more ROM, the PTA can comment that the treatment has been effective in decreasing the swelling and thus improving the ability of the elbow to move further (decreasing the severity of the impairment). See the example progress note in Figure 7–2.

3-6-92 Dx: RUE lymphedema 2° mastectomy.
   Pr: Edema RUE limiting elbow ROM with inability to feed self and groom hair using RUE.
Pt. states she is able to move her arm and use it more to help dress herself and to adjust her bed covers.
Measurements taken before and after ICP/1 hr/50 lb/30 sec on 10 sec off/supine/RUE elevated 45° to reduce edema.

	Before	After	3-4-92
Superior edge olecranon process	13"	12"	14"
3" above edge olecranon process	13.5"	12.5"	14.5"
3" below edge olecranon process	12.5"	11.5"	13.5"

All measurements read at superior edge of mark. Elbow flexion 0–95° today compared with 0–85° on 3-4-92. Observed pt. feeding self today using long-handled spoon in R hand. Needed handle extender on 3-4-92. ICP effective in reducing edema and allowing increased ROM in elbow flexion. Pt. making progress toward goal of independent feeding and grooming hair without assistive devices. Will continue ICP treatment per PT initial plan.

— Richard Student, SPTA/JimTherapist, PT Lic #1063

FIGURE 7–2   Example progress note describing a change in the impairment severity.

10-25-91 **Dx:** R CVA.
   Pr: L hemiparesis with dependent mobility in all aspects.
Pt. has been receiving PT twice a day for 3 days. Pt. able to lift buttocks with smooth motion & scoot up and down in bed 5X, roll 5X independently to L side, roll to R side with minimum assist to bring L shoulder over 5X. Pt. practiced 3X moving from sitting on edge of bed to sidelying on three pillows and returned to sitting with minimum assist to initiate sidelying to sit. Able to move from sit to stand and to return to sit from edge of bed with bed raised to highest level, SBA for cuing for even wt. bearing, 3X. Pt. ambulated from bed to bathroom to bed 3X using quad cane and moderate assist for balance and assist in advancing L leg 2X. Pt. circumducts L leg due to inability to flex knee during pre-swing. Pt. making progress toward goals of independent bed mobility, sit to stand with SBA and ambulation with quad cane and moderate assist. Will consult with PT about adding exercises for knee flexion with hip extended to improve gait next session.

— Jane Doe, PTA Lic. #2961

FIGURE 7–3 Evidence in the data information that supports the PTA's conclusion about progress toward the goal.

4-17-95 **Dx:** Bulging disc L4.
   Pr: Muscles spasms of R paraspinals limiting ability to tolerate sitting.
   S: Pt. states she still cannot sit more than 10 minutes. States she feels better if she keeps walking or moving.
   O: Massage/10 min/prone over one pillow/R paraspinal muscles L2–S1/to relax spasm followed by ice massage same area, to anaesthesia (7 min) to inhibit spasm with minimal change in muscle tone palpated. Pt. performed 10 press-up exercises and lay 5 min prone on elbows. Sat to watch body mechanics video but observed standing and pacing after 10 min. Sitting tolerance 10 min, same as last treatment session.
   A: No change in muscle tone with treatment, no change in sitting tolerance. Wondering if patient needs anti-inflammatory medication or a change in PT treatment plan.
   P: Will recommend PT re-evaluate and possible need to refer back to physician.
— Alice Alert, PTA Lic. #6240

FIGURE 7–4 An example of a progress note in which lack of progress is reported and recommendations are made.

3-19-92 **Pr:** Anterior rotation of right ilium limiting sitting and stair climbing tolerance.
Patient states she has been doing her home exercises regularly, can sit 45 minutes now, but still has pain when attempting to step up with her right leg. Reports feeling unsafe when carrying her 18-month-old daughter up the stairs. Rates her pain 7/10 before and after treatment. Pt. has been seen for three sessions. Direct contact US/1 MHz/vigorous heat/10 min/prone/right PSIS/to relax muscle spasms and prepare ligaments for mobilization. Pt. correctly performed muscle energy self-mobilization techniques to move ilium posteriorly. (See copy of instructions in chart.) Equal leg length observed supine and long sitting after US & mobilization, uneven leg length during same test before tx. Unable to palpate muscle spasms or level of PSIS due to patient's obesity. Patient correctly demonstrated her home exercises (see copy in chart), and used correct body mechanics to minimize right hip flexion when reviewing safe technique for picking up her baby. Ambulates with an antalgic limp, shorter step length and stance time on the right. Unable to step up on 7-inch stair with right leg, due to reporting too much pain. Sat with good posture, relaxed, minimal weight shifting 45 minutes watching nutrition video and waiting for her "ride." As patient was leaving the clinic, observed her climbing into her pick-up truck by stepping up with her right leg and using smooth, quick movements. This looked like it required approximately 80–90° hip flexion. Goal of 45-minute sitting tolerance met. Progress toward outcome of safe stair climbing without railing and using step-over-step pattern appears 0% in the clinic. Performance in the clinic of good sitting tolerance but poor stair climbing tolerance is inconsistent with patient's pain rating, equal leg length test, and observed performance outside the clinic. Will consult PT as to what should be done next treatment session. Pt. has two more treatment sessions scheduled.

— Puzzled Assistant, PTA Lic. #439

FIGURE 7–5 Documentation of inconsistent information in the data with reference to PT consultation.

Progress Toward Goals or Functional Outcomes

The PTA informs the reader about the patient's progress through comments about the improvement in functional abilities and in the progress toward or accomplishment of the tasks or STGs. A statement as to whether or not a goal has been met is documented in this section. The reader can find a description of the patient's functioning in the objective data that will provide evidence to support the PTA's conclusion about progress toward the goal (Fig. 7–3).

Lack of Progress Toward Goals

Lack of progress or ineffectiveness of treatment is acknowledged and comments are made as to the possible reason. The PTA may offer suggestions or indicate the need to consult the PT. Again, there should be subjective and/or objective information that provides the basis for the PTA's conclusion or opinion. Figure 7–4 is an example of a progress note reporting lack of progress and offering recommendations.

Inconsistency in the Data

Sometimes there is an inconsistency between the subjective information and the objective information. The PTA calls the reader's attention to this in the interpretation of the data content. For example, a patient may report a pain rating of 9 on a scale of 1 to 10, 10 meaning excruciating pain. The PTA may observe the patient moving about in a relaxed manner, using smooth movements with no demonstration of pain behaviors or mannerisms. This inconsistency is noted, and the PTA may want to include possible suggestions as to what to do. Again, this is a good place to recommend or refer to consultation with the PT (Fig. 7–5). *The PTA should be cautious when documenting inconsistencies, as it could be interpreted as accusing the patient of lying or faking the injury or illness.* It should be clear from the subjective and objective data that something "isn't right," and the PTA should confirm the inconsistency when interpreting the data. The inconsistency may indicate that the patient needs to be referred to another health care provider or to have the treatment plan revised.

Common Mistakes Students Make When Documenting the Interpretation of the Data Content

Too often one sees comments such as "pt. tolerated treatment well" and "pt. was cooperative and motivated." Avoid such comments unless they are *relevant* to the content of the entire progress note and are supported by the subjective and objective data. This information is better presented through descriptions of the patient's response and functional abilities.

Students commonly comment about something that is not mentioned previously in the note. Sometimes a topic is documented that appears to "come out of nowhere." Again, there must be evidence in the subjective and/or objective data to support the interpretation of the data. Figure 7–6 is an example of a note with information that is not supported by data in the note.

It is not unusual to see students' notes that do not mention the goals or provide any comments as to whether or not the patient is accomplishing the STGs. Comments tend to be only about the data that measure the impairment severity level and about the treatment procedures (Fig. 7–7).

1-17-95 **Pr:** Decreased walking tolerance due to R quad tendon repair.
   S: Pt. states eager to walk with cane, no c/o. _____
   O: tx: Respond E-stim./distal end R quad/supine/15 min/motor response/for muscle re-education. Pt. performed three sets of 15 reps of each of following strengthening exercises in supine: quad sets, terminal knee extensions, AROM hip abd./add., SLR. Pt. ambulated 150 ft from bed to down hall, tiled level surface, with single end cane in LUE, contact guard assist for sense of balance and security. _____
   A: Decreased quad strength, decreased control with knee extension ex. Concern with problem of no superior excursion with max. attempt of quad set. At max. attempt, patella is able to be shifted med. & lat. Suspicion of scarring & adhesion on R quad tendon. _____
   P: More balance work with SEC. Cont. tx 3X/week. Will consult PT about patella concerns. Pt. will see physician at 1st of next week.
   —————————————————————————————— Mary Smith, PTA Lic. #346

FIGURE 7–6   Progress note with assessment statements that are not supported by information in subjective or objective data, or both.

3-5-93 **Dx:** Fx R humerus, cast removed 3-3-93.
Pr: Limited elbow ROM with inability to reach above second button from top, face, or hair.
S: Pt. states his arm seems to be getting stronger, as he can lift a 5-lb bucket of water.

O: Elbow ROM:	before tx	after tx
flexion	40–115°	37–119°
pronation/supination	0–10° both	0–14°

All other UE ROMs WNL.

Skin that was under cast still dry and flaking, color WNL, no pressure areas evident. Wlp/102°F/20 min/RUE/to relax arm muscles, debride dry skin, and prepare for exercise. Pt. performed AROM exercises per instructions,10 reps each elbow flex/ext, forearm pronation/supination in water during last 10 min of treatment. Following wlp, pt. correctly demonstrated home exercise program to increase elbow ROM and strength (see copy in chart).

A: Moist heat and exercise effective in increasing elbow ROM.
P: Will consult PT about discontinuing whirlpool after tomorrow's session and will progress difficulty of exercises. Four more tx sessions scheduled.
— Jim Jones, SPTA/Mary Therapist, PT (Lic. #007)

FIGURE 7–7 A progress note that does not mention the goals, but confines comments only to the data that measure the impairment severity level and the treatment procedures.

SUMMARY The interpretation of the data portion of the PTA progress note provides a summary of the subjective and objective information and makes these data meaningful. Comments are made about the patient's progress and the effectiveness of the treatment. This section must *always* contain statements describing the patient's progress toward accomplishing the goals listed in the initial evaluation. It coordinates the initial evaluation with the progress notes to demonstrate PT–PTA communication, teamwork, and continuum of care. The PTA may make suggestions and report information that should be brought to the PT's attention.

All statements in this section must be supported by the subjective and/or objective information. The same rules apply that have been mentioned already regarding the subjective and objective content. The topics in this section should be organized and easy to read. All information must be relevant to the treatment plan and the patient's problem.

REFERENCE 1. American Physical Therapy Association: Guidelines for Physical Therapy Documentation. APTA, Alexandria, VA, 1995.

REVIEW EXERCISES

1. Explain why the PTA needs to interpret the significance of the subjective and objective data in the progress note.

2. List three criteria for a properly written goal or outcome.

3. Explain the PTA role in writing the goal or outcome.

4. Explain why the interpretation of the data section of the PTA progress note is the most important section to most readers of the note.

5. List the content topics to be included when interpreting the data in the PTA progress note.

6. Describe how each topic is related to the initial evaluation to demonstrate the effectiveness of the PT's treatment plan.

7. List the mistakes that students make most commonly when writing the interpretation of the data portion of the progress note.

Goals should describe an action or performance, should have measurable criteria, and should have a time frame within which the goal is expected to be accomplished. Use the LTGs and STGs in Figure 7–1. *Circle* the action or performance, *draw a line through* the time period within which the goal is expected to be accomplished, and *underline* the word or words that suggest how to measure the performance or to determine that the goal is met. The first LTG is done as an example:

Patient will (ambulate) with an assistive device and <u>minimal assist for balance to the bathroom and to meals</u> in ~~3 weeks~~.

The following STGs do not follow the criteria for them to be written correctly. They do not tell the reader much about the functional goals of the patient.

A. First, rewrite each goal so that it contains an action (verb), it can be measured, and there is a time period for accomplishing the goal.

B. Second, use your imagination and rewrite each goal so that it reads as a specific functional outcome or activity.

1. Increase right knee PROM to 0–90°.

_____

_____

_____

2. Sit on edge of bed in 3 days.

_____

_____

_____

3. Ambulate 30 ft using standard walker in 4 days.

_____

_____

_____

4. Increase strength of hip abductors from 3/5 to 4/5.

_____

_____

_____

_____

5. Decrease pain rating on pain scale from 6/10 to 3/10.

_____

_____

_____

_____

6. Return to work.

_____

_____

_____

_____

PRACTICE EXERCISE 3

Read the following progress note. _Underline_ the subjective and objective data statements that support or provide evidence for the comments in the A section.

4-17-94   **Dx:** R Colles' fracture, healed, cast removed.

Pr: Restricted ROM in wrist with inability to open doors, limited ability to grasp and pull for dressing activities.

S: Pt. reports able to put on pantyhose today without help from husband and turned bathroom doorknob to open the door.

O: Pt has been seen 2×. Pt. performed AROM exercises R forearm pronation/supination while in arm whirlpool, 110°, 20 min, to increase circulation and increase extensibility to R wrist tissues to prepare for stretching exercises. Contract–relax stretching techniques, 5 reps each, to increase pronation, supination, and wrist extension ROM, sitting with forearm supported on table. Pt. correctly demonstrated home exercise program for strengthening finger flexion, wrist flexion and extension, and forearm pronation and supination (see copy in chart). ROM today vs. 4-10-95:

	4-17-95	4-10-95
R pronation	0–50°	0–40°
R supination	0–70°	0–60°
wrist extension	0–30°	0–20°

Grip strength 20 lb today, 10 lb 4-10-95. Pt. turned door handles and opened all inside doors in the clinic using R hand, but unable to turn handle and open door to outside. Able to grasp rope on scale and pull, exerting 3-lb force (2-lb 4-10-95).

A: Strengthening and stretching treatment procedures effective in increasing strength and ROM, improving progress toward goals of independent dressing activities and ability to open all types of doors.

P: To see pt. on 4-24-95 and notify PT discharge eval. to be 4-31-95. Will work on opening outside doors next visit.

—Sally Citizen, PTA, Lic. 5631

Look at Figure 7–6. It illustrates documentation of information in the A section of this SOAP-organized note that is not mentioned in the subjective or objective sections. There is more in this note that does not constitute quality documentation. Critique the A section, and list what needs to be documented to make this a well-written progress note.

_____

_____

_____

_____

_____

_____

_____

You are on your last clinical affiliation at XXX Rehabilitation Center, where they use the SOAP format for documentation. Your patient is Jim, who has quadriplegia as a result of a spinal cord injury from a snowmobile accident. When he tries to sit, he faints because blood pools in his paralyzed legs, causing his blood pressure to drop (orthostatic hypotension). You have been working on a tilt-table treatment plan to overcome the orthostatic hypotension and to accomplish the goal of ability to tolerate the upright position for 30 minutes. The long-term goal is for Jim to be able to sit for 2 hours. It is Friday afternoon, and you are writing your weekly progress notes.

Interpret the subjective and objective data in the A section for this incomplete note. Write in black ink.

1-20-87   **Dx:** Orthostatic hypotension 2° SCI C7.

Pr: Unable to tolerate upright sitting.

S: Pt continues to c/o dizziness when he attempts sitting.

O: Pt. has had 3 sessions on the tilt table to develop tolerance for upright sitting.

First session BP dropped from 130/80 mmHg to 90/50 mmHg p̄ 10 min at 40° elevation. Today BP dropped from 130/80 mmHg ā tx to 100/60 mmHg p̄ 15 min on tilt table at 50°. BP 125/75 mmHg 5 min p̄ pt. returned to supine position.

A: _____

_____

_____

You are on your second clinical affiliation at XXX Hospital and have been working with Sally who burned her L hip. You give her whirlpool treatments daily so that the moving water will debride (i.e., clean out) the wound, and you use sterile technique to change the dressing. The goal is to promote healing of the wound so that she will be able to sit properly and begin walking. You are writing your progress note after today's treatment session. Write the interpretation of the data portion of this incomplete note. Use black ink.

11-2-85   **Pr:** Open wound due to 2nd-degree burn on L gluteus medius, not able to sit with even wt. bearing.

Pt. reports itching around edge of wound. Pt. sat in whirlpool 100°, 20 min, for wound debridement and to increase circulation for healing, sterile technique dressing change. No eschar, edges pink, 1 tsp. drainage, clear, odorless. Diameter R outer edge to L outer edge: 4 cm today compared to 4-3/4 cm 10-31-85.

CHAPTER

Writing the Content: Treatment Plan

Learning Objectives
After studying this chapter, the student will be able to:
● Compare and contrast the plan content in the evaluation with the plan content in the PTA progress note
● Discuss how the plan section incorporates the PT–PTA team approach to patient care

DEFINITION

By now the reader should see how the evaluation and progress note tell a story about the patient's physical therapy medical care. First, the patient's thoughts or contributions to the information are presented. Then the objective facts are gathered and documented. Next the information is summed up and given meaning. Finally, a **plan** is outlined in which the reader is told what is planned for the patient in the future. This information is contained in the P section in the SOAP organized note, in the E section of the DEP model, and in the second P section in the PSPG outline.

TREATMENT PLAN CONTENT

Once again, the content in the plan section is more detailed in the physical therapy evaluation than in the progress notes. APTA's *Guidelines for Physical Therapy Documentation*[1] state, "The treatment plans shall be related to the goals and should include the frequency (eg., bid, 3×/week) and duration (eg., six weeks, or 30 sessions/encounters) to achieve the stated goals" (p. 5).

Plan Content in the Evaluation

The PT outlines the treatment plans designed to accomplish the short-term goals or functional outcomes and ultimately the long-term goals or outcomes. These plans are documented in the plan section of the initial evaluation. The treatment is directed toward the physical therapy problem and includes two parts: (1) physical therapy activities or modalities that treat the impairments contributing to the patient's functional limitations and (2) practicing the functional tasks described in the short-term goals or outcomes. The PT's treatment plan will include

110

TREATMENT PLAN #1

Dx: R hip trochanteric bursitis.

Pr: Hip abductor muscle weakness and discomfort limiting tolerance for walking and stair climbing required at work.

LTG: To be able to walk from car in parking lot to office and to climb two flights of stairs without using a railing in 4 weeks for return to work.

STGs:

1. To be able to walk equivalent of two blocks with minimal hip abductor limp and 3/10 pain rating in 3 weeks.
2. To be able to climb one flight of stairs using railing and with 3/10 pain rating in 3 weeks.
3. To be able to increase hip abductor muscle strength to 5/5 in 4 weeks.

Treatment Plan:

1. Ultrasound to R trochanteric bursa, moderate heating effect, to increase circulation to decrease inflammation and discomfort.
2. Exercises, including home program, for hip abductor muscles to strengthen to grade 5/5.
3. Home program of structured, progressive walking and stair climbing activities to increase tolerance to the activities without aggravating the bursitis.

US and exercise 3X/week for 2 weeks, then 2X/week for 2 weeks with emphasis on self-management and monitoring of home programs and discontinuation of US. Pt. has appointment with physician in one month. Rehab potential is good.

TREATMENT PLAN #2

Dx: Fractures of L olecranon process and L hip.

Pr: Immobility required to allow healing causing patient to be dependent in ADLs, transfers, and ambulation so is unable to return to home.

LTG: At discharge time, patient will be able to transfer and ambulate with support for return to home.

Functional Outcomes:

1. To be able to transfer from bed <--> chair <--> toilet with SBA in 2 weeks.
2. To ambulate with platform walker for support on L from bed to bathroom, and 200 ft to be able to ambulate required distances in the home with SBA in 2 weeks.
3. To be able to ascend one step using walker and SBA to enter home in 2 weeks.

Treatment Plan:

1. Exercises to strengthen all extremities to aid transfers and ambulation. Exercise plan to include home program.
2. Training and practice for transfers from all types of surfaces as required in the home.
3. Gait training with platform walker on level tiled and carpeted surfaces and one step as required in the home.
4. Home assessment visit to clarify needs for transfer and gait training planning.
5. Educate patient and family on hip protection and safety precautions for safe functioning in the home.

Pt. to be treated bid for 2 weeks with discharge to home with support and continued physical therapy through home health agency. Rehab potential good.

TREATMENT PLAN #3

Dx: 4 weeks post fractures of L olecranon process and hip with healing in process.

Pr: Limited ROM and strength in L elbow and hip causing patient to be confined to ADLs within her home and requiring SBA.

LTG: Discharge plan is for patient to be able to transfer and ambulate independently in her home environment, and to join family for summer activities in motor home on lake.

Functional Outcomes:

1. To ambulate independently using single-end cane within the home in 3 weeks.
2. To ascend and descend stairs using single-end cane and the railing independently in 2 weeks.
3. To walk to the end of the dock using single-end cane and SBA to sit and fish in 3 weeks.
4. To climb steps into motor home using single-end cane and SBA in 3 weeks.
5. To perform home exercise program independently and accurately in 1 week.

Treatment Plan:

1. Home program of exercises to increase ROM and strength of L elbow and hip in preparation for ambulation with cane and independent ADLs.
2. Transfer and ambulation training with progression of assistive devices appropriate for safe change from platform walker to goal of single-end cane.
3. Ambulation training on grass and dock using assistive device.
4. Stair climbing training with assistive device and railing in home and into motor home.

   Home health physical therapy 3X/week for 2 weeks and decrease to 2X/week for 1 week. Rehab potential is good.

FIGURE 8–1   Three examples of documentation of treatment plans.

treatment objectives. These are written like goals, containing action words (verbs), being measurable, and having a time frame. They document the rationale for each activity or modality listed in the plan. Figure 8–1 provides three examples of documentation of treatment plans.

As the status of the patient changes and goals are met, only the *PT* may modify or change the treatment plans. These changes are documented in interim evaluations. The PTA may *not* modify the treatment plans without consulting the PT. Discharge evaluations contain the plans for any follow-up or further treatment that may be required.

When goals, functional outcomes, and treatment objectives are written correctly, the PTA can follow them to easily plan each treatment session and to measure treatment effectiveness as well as the patient's progress toward meeting the goals.

Plan Content in the Progress Note

The plan content in the PTA's progress note contains brief statements as to (1) what will be done in the next session to enable the patient to progress toward meeting the goals, (2) when the next session is scheduled, (3) what PT consultation or involvement is planned, (4) any equipment or information that needs to be ordered or prepared before the next session, and (5) the number of treatment sessions remaining before discharge.

A comment about something specific the PTA wants to be sure to do at the next session goes in the plan section. This written comment serves as a self-reminder or as a means of informing another therapist who may be treating the patient next session (e.g., "Will update written home exercise instructions next visit," "Will check skin over lateral malleolus this PM after patient has worn new AFO 6 hours").

When the PTA has commented elsewhere in the note about concerns, suggestions, or something that must be brought to the PT's attention, there should be a comment again in the plan section that the PT will be consulted or contacted (e.g., "Will consult PT about referring patient to social services"). This ensures follow-through, quality continuum of care, and PT–PTA communication. When the progress note is written by the PTA, the inclusion of a statement in the plan section that mentions the PT provides *evidence of PT–PTA teamwork.* When the situation does not require consultation or immediate communication with the PT, the PTA can demonstrate PT–PTA teamwork by referring to the PT's goals or plan in the evaluation (e.g., "Will ambulate patient on grass and curbs this PM per PT's goal in initial eval.").

When the progress note is the method for keeping track of the number of treatment sessions the patient is receiving, the number of sessions to be scheduled is reported in the plan section. The objective data may state, "Pt. has been seen for physical therapy 3×." The plan portion of the note may read, "Pt. to receive 3 more treatment sessions," "Pt. has 2 more approved visits to be scheduled," or "Pt. will return on 2-16-93, 2-23-93, and anticipate discharge on 3-1-93."

Writing the Progress Note Plan Content

The statements in the plan section of the progress note typically contain verbs in the **future tense.** The verbs describe what *will* happen between now and the next treatment session or what *will* happen at the next session.

Examples of PTA Plan Documentation

The following is a list of additional examples of plan content statements one is likely to read in a PTA's progress notes:

"Will increase weights in PRE strengthening exercises next session."
"Will discuss with PT patient's noncompliance with exercise program."
"Will consult with PT about adding ultrasound to treatment plan."
"Will notify PT that patient is ready for discharge evaluation."
"PT will see patient next session for reassessment."
"Will ambulate on stairs this PM."
"Will order standard walker to be available for treatment session on 8-4-95."
"Will have blueprints for constructing a standing table ready for home visit on 9-11-94."

SUMMARY

The plan component of physical therapy documentation addresses what will happen during subsequent treatment sessions or in the future in general. The evaluations contain the treatment plans and objectives designed by the PT to accomplish the short- and long-term goals or functional outcomes. The PTA carries out the treatment plans designed by the PT and refers to the PT when the plans need to be changed or modified. The PTA designs activities to help the patient progress within the guidelines described in the plans. The PTA documents in the plan section of the progress note what is planned for the patient at the next session(s) that will tell the reader generally how the patient will make progress toward the goal(s). The plan section may also include (1) a reminder to do something more specific, (2) statements of intent to consult with the PT regarding any concerns or suggestions that were mentioned elsewhere in the progress note, and (3) the number of treatment sessions yet to be completed. A statement in the plan section that mentions communication with the PT reinforces the PT–PTA team approach to patient care and informs the reader of this team approach.

REFERENCE

1. American Physical Therapy Association: Guidelines for Physical Therapy Documentation. APTA, Alexandria, VA, 1995, p 5.

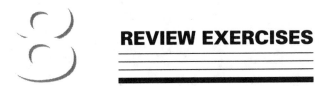

REVIEW EXERCISES

1. Discuss what the reader will find in the plan section of the PT's evaluation.

2. Describe the PTA's role in designing the treatment plan.

3. Describe the content of the plan section of a progress note.

4. Explain how the plan section of the progress note can support the PT–PTA approach to patient care.

The progress note in Practice Exercise 5 in Chapter 7 is incomplete. Finish the note by writing the plan section, stating what you will do next. Use black ink and sign the note with your legal signature and your title, SPTA.

_____

_____

_____

_____

_____

_____

_____

_____

PRACTICE EXERCISE 2

The progress note in Practice Exercise 6 in Chapter 7 is incomplete. Finish the note by writing the appropriate plan information. Use black ink and sign the note with your legal signature and your title, SPTA.

_____

_____

_____

_____

_____

_____

_____

_____

Read the treatment plans in Figure 8–1. *Circle* the activity or treatment and *underline* the measurable information. The first one is done as an example:

Ultrasound to R trochanteric bursa, moderate heating effect, to increase circulation to <u>decrease inflammation and discomfort.</u>

What are the frequencies and durations (time periods)?

CHAPTER 9

Other Documentation Responsibilities

Learning Objectives
After studying this chapter, the student will be able to:
- List other documentation responsibilities shared by the PT and PTA
- Follow proper documentation procedures when taking verbal referrals for physical therapy over the telephone
- Describe and adhere to the rule of confidentiality
- Follow proper procedures, including documentation procedures, for releasing information about a patient's condition and treatment
- Explain what to do when the patient refuses treatment
- Follow proper documentation procedures for completing and filing an incident report

The PT and PTA share other documentation responsibilities in addition to recording the physical therapy care of the patient. All clinical facilities have documentation procedures for recording telephone communications and for unusual events such as incident reports and patient refusal of treatment.

TELEPHONE COMMUNICATIONS

There are three common types of telephone conversations in which the PTA may participate that must be documented in accordance with his or her facility's procedure. These are (1) taking verbal referrals for physical therapy treatment from another health care provider, (2) receiving information about the patient from the patient or a representative of the patient, and (3) receiving inquiries about the patient's medical condition or about the physical therapy treatment from interested persons.

Referrals for Physical Therapy

Referrals for physical therapy services may be telephoned to the department by other health care providers or their staff. A physician may telephone and verbally make a referral, or the physician's nurse or even the receptionist can call in the orders. One PT may call and refer a patient to another PT with expertise in the treatment of a particular patient's condition. Another health care provider may telephone a referral because physical therapy is the more appropriate medical treatment for the condition of his or her patient. When receiving a referral over the telephone, the PTA should follow the facility's procedure for documenting the call.

Carrying a pen and notebook in your pocket at all times allows quick note taking when answering the telephone. Take notes to gather the information to document later. Each facility should have a procedure and/or form for recording telephone referrals. A copy or another similar form with the information from the call is sent to the referring provider for signature. This signature proves that the conversation and referral did take place. Typically the documentation requirements include the following:

1. Date of the call.
2. Name of the person phoning in the referral. You will know with whom to talk if questions arise later about the call or about any of the information.
3. Name of the health care provider if the call is someone other than the provider, such as the physician's receptionist.
4. Name of the PTA answering the telephone and receiving the verbal referral. Again, it is important to know who can clarify questions.
5. Details of the referral and accompanying information regarding the patient.
6. Comment regarding plans to send written verification of the telephone referral to the referring provider.
7. Comment indicating that the referral will be brought to the attention of the PT.

Information From or About the Patient

The PTA may answer the telephone when a patient or his or her family member calls to report a change in the patient's condition or ability to keep a therapy appointment. If the call is about a change in the patient's condition, the PTA may need to refer the caller to the PT or the patient's physician. If it is an emergency situation, the caller should be advised to transport the patient to the emergency room or call 911. Documentation about this call may include:

1. Date and time of the call
2. Name of the person calling
3. Name of the PTA taking the call
4. A summary of the conversation, including the response of the PTA
5. A comment regarding the apparent emotional state of the caller (tone of voice, disposition, orientation)

Requests for Information About a Patient

Often there are persons other than those providing direct patient care who have an interest in the patient's condition and treatment and who will telephone to inquire about the patient's progress. Attorneys, insurance representatives, parents of children less than 18 years of age, and other relatives, friends, and neighbors are examples of persons who might call the physical therapy department. For example, a patient who was injured while working may have lawyers, a rehabilitation manager, an insurance representative, and the employer all wanting to know about the patient's medical care. When the PTA answers the telephone and the caller asks about a patient's condition, the PTA must follow the rule of confidentiality.

The Rule of Confidentiality

All medical records and information regarding the patient's condition and treatment are confidential. Only those providing direct care to the patient have access to the information about the patient's medical care. Any individual not providing direct care to the patient must be authorized by the patient to receive information about his medical care and condition. This is an ethical principle commonly called the **rule of confidentiality.**

The patient provides this authorization by signing a **release of information form** for *each* person or by naming each person. The PTA should not provide information about the patient to anyone without first knowing whether the person is authorized to receive the in-

Release of Information Form

Patient Name_____ DOB_____
Address: _____ Social Security # _____

I authorize and request XXX Medical Rehabilitation Center to release records maintained while I was a XXX patient, disclosing information as specified below. This form may be utilized for several parties to eliminate duplicate paperwork.

PURPOSE OF REQUEST:

__X__ Insurance Reimbursement   _____ Worker's Compensation
__X__ Subsequent Treatment/Intervention on behalf of patient   _____ Damage or claim eval. by attorney
_____ Other (Specify) _____

INFORMATION TO BE RELEASED:

__X__ Eval Reports   __X__ Discharge Reports
__X__ Progress Notes   __X__ Physician Order(s)
__X__ Plan of Care   __X__ Other (Specify)_____

By placing my initials in the appropriate space, I specifically authorize XXX to include in the records released, information relating to or mentioning the following, if any:

_____ Psychological conditions   _____ Drug or alcohol abuse

RELEASE:

*1. Release to: Physician   *2. Release to: Insurance Company
   Name: Name:
   Address: Address:

*3. Release to: Employer   *4. Release to: QRC or Disability Case Manager
   Name: Name:
   Address: Address:

5. Release to: Attorney Law Firm   6. Release to: Patient
   Name: Name:
   Address: Address:

7. Release to: 8. Release to:
   Name: Name:
   Address: Address:

*When a therapist requests courtesy copies, the above parties signified by an asterisk (*) will automatically receive copies of medical records.

FIGURE 9–1   Example of a Release of Information Form (continued on next page).

formation. Once a person is determined to be authorized, the facility's procedure for releasing information should then be followed. Figure 9–1 is an example of a release of information form.

The patient's medical record is kept in a secure location, such as behind the nursing station counter or in an office, where it cannot be read easily by persons who should not have access to it. The PTA respects this rule of confidentiality by returning the patient's medical record to its proper location or by passing it on only to another authorized person. The record should never be left lying unattended on a counter or desk. Any discussion about the patient's condition must occur in private areas and only with the patient, caregivers, and those authorized to receive the information.

Any researcher who wants to gather information from the medical record must also have the patient's permission, and the researcher cannot publish or reveal the patient's name or any other descriptions that would identify the patient.

THE PATIENT'S RIGHTS The health care facility is the *legal owner* of the medical record, but the patient has the legal right to know what is in his or her medical record. The patient must follow the facility's procedure to access his or her record. This is another procedure about which the PTA should know. It usually simply involves asking the patient to sign a request form.

REVOCATION

I understand that I may revoke this authorization at any time. If I do not expressly revoke this authorization sooner, it will automatically expire 1 year from the date of this authorization; or under the following conditions:

     a.) authorization may extend beyond one year if this is a worker's compensation case.

     b.) other (specify)

COPIES

A photocopy of this authorization   ^X may   may not be accepted by you in place of the original.

SIGNATURE

Signature of patient or person   Date
authorized to sign for the patient

If signed by someone other than the patient, state how authorized

REFUSAL

I do not wish to authorize release of information to the following individual party(ies)

Name of party or parties

Signature   *Date*

FIGURE 9–1 *Continued*

PATIENT REFUSAL OF TREATMENT

As discussed in Chapter 2, the patient or a representative of the patient must consent to the treatment plan. The patient is informed of all aspects of the treatment and can give either an informal verbal consent or a formal written consent by signing an **informed consent form.** This policy and procedure ensures that the patient is not being coerced into any course of action. When the patient gives a verbal consent, the PT documents the consent in the initial evaluation. An informed consent document should contain the following[1]:

1. A description of the physical therapy problem and the proposed treatment plan written in language designed to be understood by the patient or representative of the patient
2. Name and qualifications of the PT responsible and other physical therapy personnel likely to be providing the care
3. Any risks or precautions to the treatment procedures that the patient should consider before deciding to agree to or refuse the treatment
4. An explanation of any alternative treatment that would be appropriate, including risks or precautions that need to be considered if the alternative treatment is used
5. The expected benefits of the proposed treatment plan and the expected outcomes if the physical therapy problem is not treated
6. Responsibilities of the patient or representative of the patient in the treatment plan
7. Answers to patient's questions

The patient *does have the right* to disagree with the plan or to change his or her mind later and refuse treatment. When a patient refuses treatment, there are several things the PTA can do:

1. Use active listening skills, interview, and talk with the patient to try to determine the reason for refusal. There may be a very good reason why it would not be appropriate for the patient to receive treatment at that time. I vividly remember a gentleman in a nursing home who refused therapy one day without explaining why. After spending

some time talking with him, he revealed that his dog had passed away the previous evening. This man was grieving his loss and would not have been able to concentrate on his therapy activities.

2. If there does not seem to be a reason for the refusal, make sure the patient fully understands the purpose of the treatment and the expected outcomes if the problem is not treated.
3. If the patient continues to refuse, recognize the patient's right to refuse, document this in the patient's chart, and notify the PT.

Documenting Treatment Refusal

In place of the progress note, the PTA is to document in the medical record the patient's statement of refusal and reason. The PTA is to describe his or her response and/or action and to include the statement that the PT was notified. The documentation may read as follows:

8-3-94

1:00 PM. Pt. refused treatment this PM. After being encouraged to attend at a later time, pt. stated her sister was visiting from out of state, and the only time she would be able to visit with her was this afternoon. She expected her soon and anticipated the visit would last all afternoon. Agreed to cancel treatment this PM and scheduled pt. for tomorrow AM. Will inform PT.

—Bob Smith, PTA

THE INCIDENT REPORT

Definition

An **incident** is anything that may happen to a patient, employee, or visitor that is (1) out of the ordinary, (2) inconsistent with the facility's usual routine or treatment procedure, or (3) an accident or situation that could cause an accident. All medical facilities should have a policy and procedure for the documentation of an incident, called **the incident report.** During the first or second day of internship or on a new job, the student or the newly employed PTA should read the clinic's instructions for completing and filing an incident report.

Benefits of the Incident Report

The incident report is used for risk management and legal protection. Following the incident report policy and procedure protects everyone who uses the facility (i.e., all patients, employees, and visitors) from future incidents. The procedure describes a method for providing a prompt response to medical needs, identifying and eliminating problems, and gathering and

---

THE DO'S AND DON'TS OF INCIDENCE REPORTING

1. **DO** notify your PT.
2. **DO** know your facility policy and procedure for reporting an incident.
3. **DO** write legibly and use professional terminology.
4. **DO** include the names and address of employees or visitors who know anything about the incident.
5. **DO** give the completed report to your supervising PT to route for the necessary signatures.
6. **DON'T** mention in the patient's chart that you've filed an incident report.
7. **DON'T** photocopy an incident report.
8. **DON'T** write anything in the report that implicates or blames anyone for the incident.
9. **DON'T** use incident reports for disciplinary purposes.
10. **DON'T** use the report for complaining about coworkers or other employees.
11. **DON'T** talk about the incident with noninvolved personnel. Remember *confidentiality*.
12. **DON'T** acknowledge any incident or give any information until you've checked with your PT or a supervisor.

FIGURE 9–2 Summary of the Do's and Don'ts of incident reporting. (Adapted from Documentation. In Clinical Pocket Manual. Nursing 88 Books. Springhouse Corp., Springhouse, PA, 1988, pp 135–136.)

ABC HEALTH CENTER
INCIDENT REPORT

Resident/Visitor #1 Jane Doe	Resident/Visitor #2 n/a
Address: 7700 Grand Ave. Duluth	Address:
Phone #: 628-2341 DOB 1/17/17	Phone #: DOB _____
Date: 11/21/95 Time 2:30 am/pm	Location of Incident: P.T. Dept

Description of Incident:

Pt was standing in parallel bars with PTA holding on with transfer belt, Pt performing R L/E standing exercise, she became pale and dizzy, could not walk back to chair, was lowered to floor by PTA. Never lost consciousness, felt much better once reclined. With assist of RPT was lifted into w/c

Assessment: Describe injury (if any) in detail:

Skin tear on R forearm when arm hit bar while lowering small 1.5X 2.0 open area with small amount of blood

Name/Title of All Witnesses: Mary Smith/RPT Joan Anderson/PTA	Safety Measures in Use: Transfer Belt: X Siderails: does not Restraint: use Type: _____

Intervention: None Required _____	At Facility X

Describe:

Vital signs checked and charted in nursing chart, skin tear was cleansed & protective covering in place. ROM to U/E & L L/E WFL s̄ pain! R L/E ROM within hip precaution limits s̄ pain

Resident #1

Hospitalized: Yes _____ No X	Date n/a Time _____ am/pm	Hospital n/a
Physician Name: Harvey Jones	Notified by: Dana Olson/RN Date 11/21/95 Time 3:00 am/pm	
Family Name: Robert Doe/son	Notified by: Dana Olson/RN Date 11/21/95 Time 3:15 am/pm	

Resident #2 n/a

Hospitalized: Yes _____ No _____	Date _____ Time _____ am/pm	Hospital _____
Physician Name:	Notified by: Date _____ Time _____ am/pm	
Family Name:	Notified by: Date _____ Time _____ am/pm	

FIGURE 9–3 An example of the front and back of a completed incident report. The names and situation are fictitious.

preserving information that may be crucial in litigation. The report contains information that identifies dangerous situations that either caused or could cause an injury. Risk management uses this information to change the situation so that there is no longer a risk of injury. The incident report alerts administration and the facility's lawyer and insurance company to the possibility of liability claims. It "memorializes important facts about an alleged incident that create a record for use in further investigation" (p 183).[1]

Legal Responsibility When an Incident Occurs

Only the eyewitness fills out and signs the incident report. If more than one person witnessed the incident, one of the eyewitnesses completes the report but includes the names of the other witnesses. The person documenting the incident must *follow the facility's procedure.* The incident report is completed on a form unique to the facility, but most forms used in medical facilities are similar and typically ask for the same information:

1. **Name and address of the person involved in the incident:** When the person involved is an employee or visitor, his or her home address is given. If the person is a patient, the address, date of birth, gender, admission date, and patient status before the

---

PREDISPOSING CONDITIONS

Diagnosis: Fx ⓇR hip   hypertension

Mental Status (i.e., Oriented, Alert/Confused, etc.): -alert & oriented

List pertinent medications if applicable: Tylenol   lanoxin   tenex

Follow up measures to Incident:

MD & family notified, vital signs checked every 2 hours for 12 hours

---

Was a Medical Device Involved?   ☐ Yes   ☒ No   Manufacturer's Name and Address (if Available on Equipment or Packaging):

Type _____   Model No. _____

Serial No. _____   Lot No. _____

Incident Reported By: Joan Anderson _____ Title: PTA _____

Date of Report: 11/21/95	Signature & Title of Person Preparing Report: Joan Anderson/PTA

Reviewed by DON: Virginia McDormel/Rn _____ (Signature)   Reviewed by Administrator: Mike Bond _____ (Signature)

Date: 11/22/95 ___ Charted: ☒ Yes ☐ No   Date: 11/23/95 ___

Reviewed by Medical Director: Dr Steve Jones _____ Date: 11/30/95 ___
(Signature or initials)

DO NOT WRITE BELOW THIS LINE-TO BE COMPLETED BY ADMINISTRATOR/DON

Vulnerable Adult Report Made?   ☐ Yes ☒ No

Incident Reported To (Circle as many of the following as applicable.):

Local Welfare Agency   Local Police Department   County Sheriff's Office   Office of Health Facility Complaints

Other (Explain) _____

Date Report Called in (Within 5 Days): _____   Approximate Time: _____ ☐ a.m. ☐ p.m.

Name of Person Spoken to: _____   Reported By: _____

Date Report Mailed: _____   To Whom: _____

incident.rep

FIGURE 9–3   *Continued*

incident are provided. The patient's diagnosis and physical therapy problem is recorded along with a brief summary of the care the patient has received.

2. **An objective, factual description of the incident:** The PTA completing an incident report should *not* express an opinion, should *not* blame anyone or anything, and should *not* make suggestions as to how the incident might have been prevented. The incident is to be described *as the eyewitness saw it, not* as someone else described it. There should be no secondhand information included in the report. The circumstances surrounding the incident, the condition of the affected person after the incident, and the course of action taken are described.

3. **Identification of all witnesses to the event:** The report should include addresses of the witnesses, if known, as well as identification of equipment involved by model number and manufacturer.

Each facility has a time period within which the report should be submitted. This can vary from 24 hours to 3 days after the incident. The incident *report* is not considered a medical record and is therefore placed in a file separate from the patient's medical record. *The PTA must document the incident in the patient's chart, but the incident report itself should not be mentioned.* The report is a confidential, administrative document for use in case of litigation and for risk-management review and action. Figure 9–2 summarizes the "do's and dont's" of incident reporting.[2] Figure 9–3 is an illustration of a completed incident report. The names and the situation are fictitious.

SUMMARY   The PT and PTA are responsible for numerous other documentation tasks in documenting specific events that occur during the course of a day. The PTA must know the facility's procedures for documenting various types of telephone conversations, documenting patient refusal of treatment, and completing incident reports. General descriptions of these common events and their procedures were discussed in this chapter.

REFERENCES
1. Scott, RW: Legal Aspects of Documenting Patient Care. Aspen, Gaithersburg, MD, 1994, p 123–125, 183.
2. Clinical Pocket Manual: Documentation, Nursing 88 Books. Springhouse Corp., Springhouse, PA, 1988, p 135.

REVIEW EXERCISES

1. List other documentation responsibilities shared by the PT and PTA.

2. List the information that the PTA should document when taking a verbal referral for physical therapy over the telephone.

3. Explain why the name of the caller and the name of the PTA taking the call should be documented when a referral is telephoned to the physical therapy department.

4. Describe the rule of confidentiality.

5. Discuss methods the PTA uses to adhere to the rule of confidentiality.

6. Discuss the purpose of a release of information form.

7. Discuss how the PTA should respond when the patient refuses treatment.

8. Explain how the PTA should document refusal of treatment.

9. Define an incident.

10. List what is typically included in an incident report.

11. Explain how an incident report benefits the patient, employee, and visitor.

12. Explain how an incident is documented in the patient's medical record.

Read the following scenario in which the patient refuses treatment. Document this in the form of a progress note.

You are a PTA working in a long-term care facility. You treat Janet Smith, in Room 102, daily for lower-extremity strengthening exercises, transfer training, and gait training with a walker. Ms. Smith has peripheral vascular disease with decreased circulation to her legs. She has become generally weakened due to bed rest while a small open wound on her right heel healed. You see her twice a day, and this is the third day of treatment, 11-15-95. As soon as you enter her room, she tells you she cannot have therapy today because her "right leg is too sore and swollen from being up in the wheelchair too long." You see that she is in bed, both legs elevated, T.E.D.s* (antiembolism stockings) on, and you do not observe any significant increase in edema around the lateral malleolus. She has consistently had minimal edema around the lateral malleolus. After discussing the importance of moving her legs and using her muscles to increase her circulation, you cannot convince her to participate in the therapy session. You remind her to continue doing her isometric exercises for her legs as she had been instructed when she was on bed rest, and you leave to check the nursing notes in her medical record. You see that the nurse has charted that the patient did request an increase in her usual dosage of Tylenol, which is ordered as needed. You will notify the PT and plan to see Ms. Smith tomorrow.

PROGRESS NOTE   OT_____ PT_____ SLP_____

Name:_____ Room #_____ MR# __2001__ Date_____

This therapist has observed at least every 6th treatment delivered by the assistant and deems it to be appropriate.
     __MS__

Signature_____

---

*Kendall Health Care Products, 15 Hampshire St, Mansfield, MA 02048.

Read the following scenario, which describes a situation that requires an incident report. Because you are the eyewitness, you must fill out the report. After completing the report, identify the safety lesson to be learned as a result of this incident.

You are a PTA working in a long-term care facility. You are in your patient's room working on transfer training from his wheelchair to the bed, which has wheels. Your patient is Mr. X, 75 years old, who had fractured his right hip and underwent hip repair with a prosthesis. He is allowed 40 lb of partial weight bearing and is learning to use a walker. He is alert and oriented and otherwise is in good health. The only medication he takes is Tylenol, as needed. The plan is for him to be discharged to his home, where he lives with his 70-year-old wife. It is Friday, December 1, 1995, 10:20 AM. Mr. X stands from the wheelchair and proceeds to do a

(continued on page 132)

INCIDENT REPORT

Resident/Visitor #1:	Resident/Visitor #2:
Address:	Address:
Phone #: DOB_____	Phone #: DOB_____
Date: Time____ am/pm	Location of Incident:

Description of Incident:

Assessment: Describe injury (if any) in detail:

Name/Title of All Witnesses:	Safety Measures in Use:
	   Transfer Belt:_____
	   Siderails:_____
	   Restraint:_____ Type:_____

Intervention: None Required _____   At Facility _____

Describe:

Resident #1

Hospitalized: Yes___ No___	Date_____ Time_____am/pm	Hospital_____
Physician Name:	Notified by: Date_____Time____am/pm	
Family Name:	Notified by: Date_____Time____am/pm	

Resident #2

Hospitalized: Yes___ No___	Date_____ Time_____am/pm	Hospital_____
Physician Name:	Notified by: Date_____Time____am/pm	
Family Name:	Notified by: Date_____Time____am/pm	

PREDISPOSING CONDITIONS

Diagnosis:

Mental Status (i.e., Oriented, Alert/Confused, etc.):

List pertinent medications if applicable:

Follow-Up Measures to Incident:

Was a Medical Device Involved? ☐ Yes ☐ No Manufacturer's Name and Address (If Available on Equipment or Packaging):

Type_____ Model No. _____

Serial No. _____ Lot No. _____

Incident Reported By:_____ Title:_____

Date of Report:	Signature & Title of Person Preparing Report:

Reviewed by DON:_____
    (Signature)

Date:_____ Charted: ☐ Yes ☐ No

Reviewed by Administrator:_____
    (Signature)

Date:_____

Reviewed by Medical Director:_____ Date:_____
    (Signature or Initials)

DO NOT WRITE BELOW THIS LINE - TO BE COMPLETED BY ADMINISTRATOR/DON

Vulnerable Adult Report Made? Yes ☐ No ☐

Incident Reported To (Circle as many of the following as applicable.):

Local Welfare Agency   Local Police Department   County Sheriff's Office   Office of Health Facility Complaints

Other (Explain)_____

Date Report Called In (Within 5 Days):_____

Name of Person Spoken to:_____

Date Report Mailed:_____

Approximate Time:_____ ☐ a.m. ☐ p.m.

Reported By:_____

To Whom:_____

(continued from page 130)

standing pivot transfer with the walker to get into bed. You have the transfer belt on him and you are standing on his right side. As he turns, his left knee buckles and he starts to fall. You guide him down onto the bed, but the bed rolls back and you must lower the patient to the floor. You rest his head and trunk in your lap, call for help, and notice that his legs are positioned straight in front of him. He denies having pain in his right hip or leg, but does complain of pain in his right buttock. He is nervous and anxious. The nurse, Jane Doe, and a nursing assistant, Tom Jones, hear you and come running. With their help, you are able to lift Mr. X up and into bed. The resident in orthopedic surgery, Dr. Young, happens to be in the building. He is called and is able to examine Mr. X immediately. He doesn't think there has been any damage to his hip and believes the buttock pain may be due to bumping against the side rail as he was lowered to the floor. Nursing will monitor the skin condition and his pain complaints, and Mr. X will rest in bed for the remainder of the day.

Safety lesson: _____

_____

Documentation Summary: Study Guide*

The previous nine chapters in this book have objectives, review exercises, and practice exercises to help the reader learn the information. This chapter presents important points from the book in an outline format for quick reference and for use as a study guide.

I. Introduction to Documentation

A. Definition

    1. A legal record of the patient's medical care from admission to discharge.

    2. Written proof that authenticates the care given to the patient.

    3. A written record holding the caregiver accountable for the quality of the care and for the cost placed on that care.

    4. The rationale that supports the medical necessity of the treatment.

B. The evolution of PT and PTA responsibilities.

    1. Historically, changes in physician referral influenced changes in PT and PTA treatment and documentation responsibilities.

      a. Referrals used to read like a prescription, telling the therapist exactly what to do. Therapist a technician, providing physical therapy treatments.

      b. With education by PTs, referrals changed to read "evaluate and treat."

        (1) PT needed evaluation skills to problem solve and to identify the patient's musculoskeletal problems that could be treated with physical therapy.

        (2) PT documented the physical therapy evaluations.

        (3) First PTA school opened in 1967. The PTA is the technical health care provider who provides physical therapy treatments under the direction and supervision of the PT.

      c. Direct access in Nebraska since 1957, in California 1968, in Maryland 1979; direct access legislation pending in other states. Direct access allows the consumer to seek physical therapy services without a referral from the physician.

        (1) PT has additional responsibility to recognize a patient's signs and symptoms that are not treatable by physical therapy and to refer the patient to more appropriate health care providers.

        (2) PTA responsibility increased to team up with the PT in assessing the patient's response to treatment.

---

* Review questions are not applicable for this chapter. The reader will find practice exercises after the study guide.

2. The establishment of Medicare (Health Insurance for the Aged and Disabled Act) in 1965.
   a. Documentation standards that required accountability for treatment dollars requested by the caregiver.
   b. Stage set for documentation standards and criteria established by federal and state governments and various agencies.
3. Limited dollars available for high health care costs.
   a. The *major* factor influencing the treatment and documentation responsibilities of the PT and PTA at present.
   b. Most effective and efficient PT treatments must be identified and used.
   c. Insurance companies scrutinize medical records to identify and support the health care providers that give quality medical care as efficiently as possible and at a reasonable cost.
   d. Documentation must be done properly to reflect effective and efficient care.
4. Effectiveness of physical therapy care is measured in terms of how well the patient can function in his or her environment and is documented in the description of the patient's functional abilities.

C. Role of documentation in ensuring quality of care.
   1. Good communication among caregivers: The method by which all the patient's health care providers communicate with one another.
   2. Basis for reimbursement decisions. The third-party payer will not reimburse for treatment procedures that do not seem appropriate or effective.
   3. Information or data for research activities (e.g., physical therapy research designed to determine efficacy of physical therapy treatment procedures).
   4. Documentation standards and criteria defined by the following:
      a. Federal government (Medicare).
      b. State government (Medicaid, Medical Assistance, Workers' Compensation, state physical therapy practice acts).
      c. Professional agencies (e.g., APTA).
      d. Accrediting agencies (e.g., JCAHO, CARF).
      e. The individual health care facility.
   5. Follow the documentation standards by *following the facility's procedures*.

II. Documentation Content

A. Information in the medical record is grouped into six general content categories.
   1. **Data:** All information about the patient that relates to (1) why the patient is seeking medical help and (2) the patient's response to the medical care provided.
      a. Subjective data: Information gathered through an interview of the patient or a representative of the patient. Information that is *told* to the caregiver.
      b. Objective data: Information gathered by the health care provider through an examination or evaluation. Information that can be measured, reproduced, or observed by another health care provider with the same training.
   2. **The problem requiring medical treatment:** Data are analyzed, and the analysis results in the identification of the problem(s) that require medical treatment.
      a. Medical diagnosis: Identification of a systemic disease or disorder determined by the physician's examination.
      b. PT evaluates the patient and determines the physical therapy problem.
      c. Physical therapy problem: Neuromusculoskeletal dysfunction that interferes with the patient's ability to function in his or her environment.
      d. Incorporates the patient's impairment with his or her functional limitations.
   3. **Treatment plan or action:** Plan of action to treat the problems.
      a. Outlined in the medical record.
      b. Must give patient information about the treatment plan, and patient must give informed consent before the plan is initiated.
   4. **Goals, functional outcomes, or purpose for the treatment plans** documented.

a. Give direction to the medical care and a means of measuring the effectiveness of the treatment.

b. Goals must be functional goals.

c. Goals must be the patient's goals.

5. **Record of administration of the treatment plan:** Includes the daily or weekly progress notes.

6. **Treatment effectiveness**

a. Information that records the interpretation of the patient's response to the treatment.

b. Most important information in the medical record. Answers the question, *"Is the treatment appropriate and effective?"*

B. Documentation responsibilities.

1. PT responsible for documenting the evaluations.

2. Primary documentation responsibility for the PTA is writing the progress notes. The PTA shares this task with the PT.

C. The physical therapy evaluations.

1. The PTA *can* assist the PT in performing an evaluation.

a. The PTA can take notes for the PT.

b. The PTA can assist in gathering subjective data.

c. The PTA may perform tests in which he or she has been trained, such as goniometry, manual muscle testing, taking vital signs, and measuring girth.

2. The PTA *cannot* interpret the evaluation data, identify the physical therapy problem, design or modify the treatment plan, or set treatment goals.

3. The PTA carries out the PT's treatment plan and assists the patient in accomplishing the treatment goals.

4. There are three types of physical therapy evaluations:

a. Initial evaluation: Performed the first time the PT sees the patient. *The PTA cannot treat a patient who has not undergone a PT's initial evaluation.*

b. Interim evaluations: These are performed periodically during the course of the physical therapy treatment to measure the patient's progress and to change or modify the treatment plan as indicated. The PTA writes progress or interim *notes,* but the PT documents interim *evaluations.*

c. Discharge evaluation: This is the final note about the patient, summarizing the treatment that was provided, concluding the degree of effectiveness of the treatment, and recommending further care if needed. The PT documents the discharge evaluation.

5. The PTA may write a discharge summary.

a. The information is only a summary of the treatment provided and a description of the patient's status at discharge.

b. The summary should not include an interpretation of the information or recommendations for further care after discharge.

c. The PTA discharge summary cannot be the final note about the patient's care in the chart.

III. Organization of the Content

A. The information in the medical record is typically organized according to the disciplines providing the medical care, the patient's problems, or a combination.

1. The SOMR is organized according to the medical services the patient is receiving.

2. The POMR is organized according to the list of problems being treated by the health care providers.

B. Organization of the documentation content in the medical record can be in a variety of formats, each with its own logical arrangement of components.

1. At present, SOAP organization is the most common format for arranging the information.

a. S stands for subjective, and this section contains the subjective data.

    b. O stands for objective, and this section contains the objective data.

    c. A stands for assessment, and this section contains the interpretation of the data, identification of the problems, and goals.

    d. P stands for plan, and this section contains the treatment plan.

2. PSPG is a format often used in progress notes that accompany a SOAP-organized evaluation.

    a. The P section contains the statement of the patient's problem(s).

    b. The S section contains the status of the patient at the time of the note. It includes the subjective and objective data.

    c. The P section contains the plan for future treatment sessions.

    d. The G section contains the goals, with statements about progress toward the goals, any goals accomplished, and any new goals set.

3. DEP is a documentation format in the process of being developed.

    a. D stands for data, and this section contains both the subjective and objective data.

    b. E stands for evaluation, and this section contains the interpretation of the data, the problems, and the treatment plan.

    c. P stands for performance goals, and this section identifies the functional goals that the treatment is designed to accomplish. The goals include a time frame within which the goal is expected to be reached.

4. All the models for organizing the documentation content have a common thread. The PTA can adapt to any model when writing progress notes by following these guidelines:

    a. Introduce the progress note with a listing or statement that tells the reader the physical therapy problem(s) about which the note is written.

    b. Next, provide the subjective data and objective data. Compare it or relate it to the data in the PT's evaluation.

    c. Discuss the meaning of the data as it relates to treatment effectiveness and the patient's progress toward accomplishing the goals listed in the PT's evaluation.

    d. Discuss the plan for future treatment sessions and involvement of the PT.

C. The content can be presented in a variety of formats.

1. Computerized documentation.

2. Flow charts and checklists: These are used mainly by hospitals, rehabilitation centers, and nursing homes.

3. Letter, typically to the physician: This is used by private practice outpatient clinics.

4. The IEP: This is used in schools.

5. The cardex format: This is used within physical therapy departments to record the current treatment procedures for the patient. Another PT or PTA should be able to duplicate the treatment by following the information written on the cardex.

6. Medicare forms: Medicare has standardized forms for documenting patient status and for seeking recertification for further treatment.

IV. Writing the Content: Guidelines

A. The focus is on writing the progress note

1. The progress note is the record of the treatment procedures administered and their effectiveness.

2. Typically, the progress note is written daily when the patient's condition is acute and weekly if the condition is more chronic. If the patient is seen intermittently (e.g., once a week, twice a week, three times a week), a note is written after each therapy visit.

3. The content of a progress note must include the following:

    a. Specific treatment provided, purpose, and the patient's response to each treatment procedure.

    b. Equipment provided or sold to the patient and any written instructions given to the patient.

   c. Patient status, progress toward goals, or lack of progress written in *functional terms*.

4. The organization of the content of the progress note must be in a form the facility uses.

5. The medical diagnosis and/or the physical therapy problem may introduce the progress note.

B. There are *principles and guidelines for documenting in a legal record* that must be followed by everyone writing in a medical record. Write as if writing a letter to a jury or to a lawyer, and follow the legal guidelines.

1. Be accurate. *Never falsify the information.*

2. Be brief. Sentences should be short and concise. The information should be relevant.

   a. Abbreviations should be used minimally or not at all.

   b. Abbreviations can be misunderstood, and that can be dangerous.

3. Be clear.

   a. When describing the patient's function, the words should "paint a picture of the patient" so that the reader can "see" the patient in his or her mind.

   b. Handwriting should be legible. Sloppy handwriting suggests sloppy thinking and work.

   c. Punctuation, grammar, and spelling should be correct. It demonstrates that you are careful not to make mistakes.

4. Date and sign all entries.

   a. Use full legal signature.

   b. Place the initials of your title after the signature.

   c. Write your license number after your title initials. This identifies that the physical therapy treatment was provided by a qualified, trained physical therapy provider.

5. Use black ink. This guideline may change.

6. Do not allow opportunity for the record to be changed or falsified.

   a. Do not use erasable pens.

   b. Do not erase errors. Cross them out with one line, write the date and your initials above the error.

   c. Do not leave lines blank. Draw a line through any blank lines or large spaces.

   d. Be timely. Carry a notebook and pen in your pocket to take quick notes for accurate documentation later.

V. Writing the Content: Subjective Data

A. Subjective data consist of information about the patient and the patient's condition that is *told* to the health care provider by either the patient or a representative of the patient.

1. Subjective data in the progress note must be *relevant* to the patient's physical therapy problem and treatment.

   a. While working with the patient, the PTA uses active listening, which includes analytic listening, directed listening, attentive listening, and exploratory listening.

   b. Relevant information is grouped in the categories of medical history, environment, emotions or attitudes, goals or functional outcomes, unusual events or chief complaints, response to treatment, and level of functioning.

2. The patient's complaints that cause him or her to seek medical help are the symptoms of the patient's condition, and the symptoms are subjective data.

B. Organizing and writing the subjective content.

1. The subjective data can be organized or grouped according to the content categories listed in V.A.1.b. when there are detailed data to record.

2. The progress note does not have to contain subjective data. It is written only if the information is relevant to the effectiveness of the treatment session(s).

3. Guidelines for writing subjective data:

      a. Use verbs such as states, reports, denies, says, and describes.

      b. Quote the patient directly to document clearly the patient's confusion, denial, attitude toward therapy, and use of abusive language.

      c. When information is provided by someone other than the patient, document who provided the information.

C. Information about pain is included in the subjective data section.

  1. Pain is perceived and described by the patient.

  2. It is best described in some form of a pain profile.

      a. Pain scale, usually numerical.

      b. Checklist of descriptive words.

      c. Body drawing and color codes.

  3. Pain profiles are always located in the subjective data section of the progress note.

VI. Writing the Content: Objective Data

A. Objective data consist of information about the patient's condition that is gathered by examination, testing, evaluation, and observation.

  1. The information can be measured, reproduced, and/or observed by another health care provider with the same training.

  2. The objective data include the signs of the patient's condition.

  3. Visual or tactile observations made by the PTA are objective data when another PT or PTA would see or feel the same information.

B. Organizing and writing the objective data.

  1. The organization of the content should be such that the information flows from one topic to the next.

  2. Group the content into categories.

      a. Results of measurements and tests.

      b. Description of patient's functioning.

      c. Description of treatment provided.

  3. Writing the objective content guidelines:

      a. Repeat tests and measurements that were taken during the initial evaluation to assess the patient's response to treatment.

      b. Document the results in such a way that the reader can easily compare them with the results in the initial or previous evaluations or notes.

      c. Use words to describe the patient performing a function so that the reader can picture the patient's functioning in the reader's mind. Paint a picture of the patient functioning.

      d. Write a description of the treatment provided in enough detail that another PT or PTA could read the description and duplicate the treatment. This detailed description can be found in the progress note and/or cardex in the physical therapy department.

      e. Include the purpose for each treatment procedure and the patient's response to each treatment procedure. This information will be useful for researching the most effective treatment procedures.

      f. Include a copy of any written information given to the patient.

      g. Talk about any equipment provided or sold to the patient.

C. Common mistakes students make when writing objective data.

  1. Writing what *they* did and not what the *patient* did.

  2. Rambling or failing to organize the information by topic.

VII. Writing the Content: Problems, Goals or Functional Outcomes, and Treatment Effectiveness

A. Problems, goals or functional outcomes, and treatment effectiveness constitute the interpretation of the data.

  1. This documentation content is most commonly considered assessment information and is included in the A section of the SOAP note.

  2. Answers the "so what?" question a reader might ask after reading the data.

     3. Gives meaning to the data.

     4. Provides the rationale for the necessity of the treatment.

B. Interpretation of the data in the PT evaluation.

     1. Identifies the physical therapy problem based on the data.

     2. Lists the LTGs and STGs.

     3. Lists functional outcomes when goals are not used. Goals or outcomes:

       a. Describe the action.

       b. Have measurable criteria that determine their accomplishment.

       c. Have a time period within which they are expected to be accomplished.

C. Interpretation of the data in the progress note.

     1. Comments about the effectiveness of the treatment procedures and the treatment plan as a whole.

     2. Comments about the patient's progress toward accomplishment of the short- and ultimately long-term goals and functional outcomes.

     3. Comments about lack of progress and any suggestions or recommendations to be discussed with the PT.

     4. *All comments should be supported with evidence in the subjective and objective data.*

     5. Note whether there is inconsistency between the subjective and objective data.

     6. *Always relate the interpretation of the data to the information in the PT's initial evaluation.*

D. Common mistakes students make when interpreting the data.

     1. Vague comments about the patient's condition or progress.

     2. Comments that are not supported by evidence in the subjective or objective data.

     3. Tendency to forget to talk about the progress toward the goals or functional outcomes.

VIII. Writing the Content: Treatment Plan

A. The plan content in the PT's initial evaluation contains the treatment plan and objectives set by the PT. The plan is:

     1. Designed to accomplish the goals or outcomes.

     2. Directed toward eliminating or minimizing the impairment.

     3. Includes practicing the functional tasks required to accomplish the functional outcomes.

     4. Cannot be modified by the PTA.

B. The plan content in the progress note tells the reader what the PTA will do at the next treatment session or between one session and the next.

     1. Indicate when the next session will be and/or how many more sessions are scheduled.

     2. Include a comment that demonstrates the PT's involvement. It should reinforce the PT–PTA team approach to physical therapy patient care.

     3. Use verbs in the future tense.

IX. Other Documentation Responsibilities

A. Documenting telephone conversations.

     1. Verbal referral for physical therapy.

       a. Note data about the patient.

       b. Note name of the caller and name of the PTA taking the call.

       c. Note date and time of the call.

       d. Note that the referral will be brought to the PT's attention.

       e. Send a written copy of the information to the caller for signature.

     2. When the patient or representative of the patient calls to report a change in the patient's condition, the PTA may:

       a. Refer the caller to the PT.

       b. Refer the caller to the patient's physician.

       c. Advise the caller to take the patient to the ER or to call 911.

      d. Document in the patient's chart the date and time of the call, the name of the caller, and the PTA taking the call, as well as a description of the conversation including the action taken by the PTA.

  3. When someone calls asking about the condition of the patient:

      a. Only the persons directly providing patient care are permitted to have access to the patient's medical record. This is the *rule of confidentiality*.

      b. The patient can authorize other persons to have access to his or her medical information by signing a release of information form for *each* person.

      c. The PTA cannot release any information about the patient to any unauthorized person.

      d. Good rule: When the PTA is unsure whether he or she should answer the caller's question, the PTA should *refer the caller to the PT*.

      e. The PTA is to discuss the condition of the patient only in private and only with authorized persons.

B. Patients' rights and documentation.

  1. The patient has the right to know what is written in his or her medical record.

      a. The medical record is owned by the medical facility.

      b. The patient typically signs a form to access his or her medical record.

  2. The patient has the right to consent to treatment.

      a. The patient is informed of all the details of the treatment plan.

      b. The patient consents either verbally or formally (in writing) to the treatment plan before it is initiated.

      c. Formal consent is made by the patient's signing an informed consent form with the PT (*not the PTA*) witnessing the signature.

      d. The verbal or formal consent is documented in the PT's initial evaluation.

  3. The patient has the right to refuse treatment.

      a. The patient may refuse a treatment session or refuse to continue treatment.

      b. Use active listening skills, talk with the patient, and try to determine the reason for the refusal.

      c. Be sure the patient understands the purposes of the treatment and the consequences of not being treated.

      d. Refer the patient to the PT.

      e. The PTA may need to allow the patient to refuse.

      f. Document the conversation in the patient's chart.

C. Documenting the incident report.

  1. An incident is anything out of the ordinary that happens to a patient, employee, or visitor. It is:

      a. Not part of the facility's usual routine, treatment procedures, or functioning of the equipment.

      b. An accident or something that could cause an accident.

  2. The incident is documented in the facility's incident report form.

      a. The form must be: Documented within the time period after the incident as specified in the facility's procedure.

      b. Written by the eyewitness only.

      c. Written factually, as it happened, including time, location, name of person involved, names and addresses of eyewitnesses, conditions of the environment, equipment, condition of the person involved before and after the incident, action(s) taken.

      d. Without opinions, blames, or suggestions.

      e. Completed and signed by the eyewitness to the incident.

  3. The incident report is designed to:

      a. Inform risk management of hazards and potential hazards that can be corrected.

      b. Alert administration, lawyers, and insurance company representatives of the possibility of a liability claim.

      c. Protect the patient, employee, and visitor.

Name: Mrs. S.   **Physician:** Dr. R.
Facility: XXXX Nursing Home   **Date:** 4-22-93

Dx: Left humerus and left hip fracture.

Subjective: Pt. states she had fallen on bricks while at the St. Patrick's Day parade on 3-17-93. She saw Dr. R. on 4-21-93 when he removed the immobilizer and ordered the start of physical therapy. States she lives in senior housing where there are no steps for her to climb, has been independent, drove her car, and did all her household chores, cooking, and self care; wants to return to independent living. Past medical Hx: fractured R hip 12 years ago and was back to normal, everyday living without the use of an assistive device. Mastectomy on left 30 years ago and has swelling and pain in LUE since. Arthritis in both hips. Ccs: bladder infection, dizziness when first up in sitting, and nervousness and apprehension about therapy. Nursing reports pt. has not been up out of bed much for the past month due to her refusing.

Objective: Palpation revealed no tenderness to the lower extremity or the upper extremity. Pt. did have minimal swelling in the left ankle and mod. to max. swelling in the LUE at wrist and elbow (measurements not taken).

ROM (measured in supine)

	Active	Passive
L shoulder flexion	0° c/o pain	0–95°
L should abduction	0–55°	0–90°
L shoulder ER	0°	0–12°
L shoulder IR	WNL	WNL
L elbow flexion	WNL	WNL

Wrist and finger flexion slightly decreased by swelling. L knee flexion in supine 0–65°. MMT— L hip flexors 5-/5, L quads 4+/5, L hamstrings 5-/5, L shoulder flexors 2/5, L shoulder abductors 2/5, L shoulder IR & ER 4/5. Transfers —Able to perform standing pivot transfer wheelchair to mat with mod. assist for balance; pt. uses only RUE. Holds LUE in somewhat guarded position and unable to bear much wt. on LLE. Sit to supine with min. assist for control in lowering trunk; able to lift LLE. Supine to sit with mod. assist for raising herself (unable to use LUE to help), sit to stand with standby assist for balance. Independent stand to sit with LLE extended due to decreased knee flexion, but pt. sits on edge of bed, leans backward, and complains of dizziness. Ambulation—Pt. ambulated in hall on tiled surface with rolling walker, SBA for balance, 25 ft, wt. bearing as tolerated on left. L shoulder was depressed, as pt. was not bearing wt. on LUE.

Physical Therapy Problem: Decreased ROM, strength, and mobility secondary to a left humerus and left hip fracture requiring dependent transfers and ambulation.

Goals:

LTG: To return to independent living and to return to her previous lifestyle.

STGs:
1. To increase strength to at least 4/5 in all LUE muscles to aid in transfers and ambulation in 2 months.
2. To increase ROM to WFL for all shoulder, hip, and knee motions to aid in transfers and ambulation in 1 month.
3. To perform independent transfers from bed, toilet, various heights chairs and ambulation with assistive device on tiled, carpeted, and sidewalk level surfaces in 2 months.
4. To perform home exercise program independently and accurately in 2 weeks.

Treatment Plan:
1. AROM and gentle stretching exercises to all shoulder, hip, and knee motions to increase ROM for transfer and ambulation activities.
2. Strengthening exercises for all UE muscles, including home program to aid transfers and ambulation.
3. Gait training with assistive device on tiled and carpeted level surfaces and on sidewalk.
4. Transfer training from bed <--> chair <--> toilet and from various heights and types of chairs and couches for independent functioning in the home.
5. Home assessment visit to clarify needs for transfer and ambulation training planning.

Pt. to be treated bid for 3 weeks and decrease to 1X/day, 5X/week for 5 weeks. Anticipate discharge to independent living at home in 2 months. Rehab potential good.

— Mary Therapist, PT (Lic. #)

FIGURE 10-1   A physical therapy initial evaluation.

5-18-93 **Dx:** L humerus & L hip Fx.
      Pr: Dependent transfers, ambulation, and limited knee ROM.
      S: Pt. states she sat in the lounge chair in her room last night without needing to extend her L leg because she could bend her knee more now; nurses upset with her because she walked Ⓘ in room with standard walker last night. Denies having dizziness._____
      O: Contract-relax stretching/3 sets/4 reps/to gain L knee flexion/sitting in lounge chair. After tx, AROM L knee flexion 0–75°, PROM 0–80°, measured goniometry sitting (0–65° in initial eval.). Observed pt. Ⓘ sit to stand from lounge chair using R hand in center of walker, L hand on arm of chair. Ambulated min. assist for pt. sense of security, wide-base quad cane to protect LLE, lounge chair to nursing station (@ 50 ft), tiled surface, rest, and ambulated back. Needed assist for mild loss of balance recovery 1X. Observed pt. ambulate Ⓘ, standard walker, chair to bathroom, stand to sit, sit to stand from toilet, ambulate room to dining room (@ 100 ft), partial wt. bearing L._____
      A: Improved knee flexion allows easier transfers from low chair and toilet. Progress toward STGs #2 and #3 in initial evaluation is 75%. Ready to be allowed independent ambulation with walker in room and on nursing floor._____
      P: Will notify PT of Ⓘ amb. status with walker so nursing can be notified. Will continue to progress pt. with quad cane and add ambulating on carpeting tomorrow AM._____
                                     — Jim Doe, PTA

FIGURE 10-2   A progress note relating to the initial evaluation in Figure 10–1.

    4. The incident report is confidential.
      a. The report is placed in a special file.
      b. The incident is documented in the patient's chart.
      c. *Make no reference to the incident report in the chart, and do not put the report in the chart.*

SUMMARY

The PTA is responsible for complete, accurate, and proper physical therapy documentation in the patient's medical record. All documentation should be clear to anyone who reads the chart, regardless of the reader's training. The PTA provides documentation primarily in the progress note, which provides evidence that the PT's treatment plan is being carried out and that the plan is effective in improving the patient's level of functioning in his or her environment.

The theories and skills described in this text are illustrated in the PT's initial evaluation in Figure 10–1. The PTA's progress note relating to the initial evaluation is shown in Figure 10–2.

GUIDELINES FOR CRITIQUING THE PROGRESS NOTE

As you read and critique a progress note, look first at the organization to see if the writer:
1. Introduced the progress note with a listing or statement that tells the reader the physical therapy problem(s) about which the note is written.
2. Placed the subjective and objective data first.
3. Compared or related these data to the data in the PT's initial evaluation.
4. Discussed the meaning of the data in terms of treatment effectiveness and progress toward accomplishing the functional goals listed in the PT's evaluation.
5. Discussed the plan for future treatment sessions and involvement of the PT.

Next, look more specifically at each content area.

1. Were legal guidelines followed?
    Black ink or typed?
    Legible?
    Error crossed out with one line?
    Error dated and initialed?
    Note dated?
    Complete legal signatures with titles?
    Lines drawn through long blank spaces?
2. Subjective data:
    Are they information *told* to the therapist?
    Are they information *relevant* to the treatment session?
    If pain is documented, is it in the subjective data section?

3. Objective data:

Is there enough information about the treatment provided so that another therapist could duplicate the treatment?

Is the purpose of the treatment documented?

Is the target tissue or treatment area identified?

Is there a description about how the patient performs functional activities?

Can the reader clearly visualize the patient's performance; does the note paint a picture of the patient?

Does the note describe what the PT or PTA observed?

Was a copy of the written instructions or information given to the patient put in the chart?

Are measurements consistent with the measurements in the initial evaluation?

Are measurements related or compared to previous measurements?

4. Interpretation of the data:

Does this section answer the "so what?" question? Does it give meaning to the data?

Does the information summarize the subjective and objective data?

Are there statements about the patient's progress toward accomplishing the STGs and LTGs listed in the initial evaluation?

Are there statements about patient's progress toward accomplishing the functional outcomes listed in the initial evaluation?

Are any concerns or suggestions mentioned?

Are there statements that are not supported by the subjective and/or objective information?

5. Plan:

Does the information relate to what will happen next?

Is there information about the number of treatment sessions scheduled, the number remaining, and anticipated discharge?

Is there reference to the PT's plan, the PT's initial evaluation, working with the PT, or consulting the PT?

Overall, does the note describe quality physical therapy care in such a manner that anyone reading the note will understand the information?

Copy the statements in the following narrative PTA progress notes under the appropriate categories.

PROGRESS NOTE 1

3-10-88

Pt. is disoriented. She states, "It is Christmas and I don't have my shopping done." Observed pt. scratching at her wound dressings. Pt. has a decubitus over L lat. malleolus interfering with ability to wear proper shoe for ambulation. Wound dressing half off upon arrival to dept. Wound measures 3 cm horizontally across outer edge to outer edge (4 cm initial eval.), loose necrotic tissue, no drainage. Foot whirlpool 104°F, loose tissue dislodged, and dressings changed. Will consult PT re: designing wrap over bandage to keep pt. from pulling dressing loose. 50% progress toward goal of clean, healing wound to prepare for ambulation.—Sue Smith, PTA

Problem Statement:

Pr: _____

_____

Subjective Data:

S: _____

_____

_____

Objective Data:

O: _____

_____

_____

Interpretation of the Data:

A: _____

_____

_____

Plan Statement(s):

P: _____

PROGRESS NOTE 2

2-10-90

     Pt. ambulated 3× the length of the // bars (about 30 ft) c̄ min. assist for sense of security, with verbal cues for posture and heel–toe stepping. He needs max. assistance for sit ↔ stand for strength to get up and for control when sitting down. Gluteus maximus and quads 3/5. Major mm groups in LEs 3/5 to 4/5 strength range. Pt. is not independent in ADL due to muscle weaknesses. Pt. states he wants to go home. Maximum assist for transfer bed ↔ commode ↔ w/c. Will continue to work to ↑ mm strength and try sliding board transfers this PM. Pt. demonstrated 3 reps each of LE strengthening exercises to be performed in the ward with wife's help (see copy in chart). Pt.'s wife says she cannot care for pt. at home. Pt. is 82 years old c̄ terminal cancer.

Problem Statement:

Pr. _____

Subjective Data:

S: _____

_____

_____

Objective Data:

O: _____

_____

_____

Interpretation of the Data:

A: _____

_____

_____

Plan:

P: _____

_____

_____

Place "Pr" next to statements that are physical therapy problems, "SD" next to subjective data statements, "OD" next to objective data statements, "ID" next to statements that interpret the data, and "P" next to plan statements.

_____ Pt. reports pain relief several hours after treatment.

_____ Performed Codman's exercises with 2-lb wt. to distract shoulder.

_____ Electrode placed 2 inches above R elbow crease line.

_____ R hemiplegia with spasticity and dependence for transfers and ambulation.

_____ Will instruct in proper stair climbing next session.

_____ Missed 2 of his last 5 treatment sessions due to illness one day and refusal the other.

_____ C/o pain in RLE.

_____ Recommended family install railing on wall along stairs for safety.

_____ Goal met for child to roll side-lying to supine and prone 1/3 trials at least 3× in 2 months to improve mobility.

_____ Had terrible headache last night.

_____ Will await further orders from physician.

_____ Pt. able to demonstrate home exercise program with good form.

_____ Pain intensity increased from 5 to 6/7.

_____ Requires moderate assist to get up from w/c and to lift legs back into bed.

_____ States he needs to lift a maximum of 70 lb from floor to conveyor belt.

_____ Performed 10 reps of UED1 exercises on the R using red Thera-Band* and 20 reps of same exercise on the L with blue Thera-Band.

_____ Ambulated with forceful knee hyperextension during stance phase.

_____ My goal is to play golf.

_____ Atrophy of quads and gastrocs limiting ability to manage stair climbing.

_____ Will take standard walker to patient's home next visit.

_____ Wrist flexors 3/5, extensors 2/5 strength.

_____ Mother stated child rolled supine to prone last night.

_____ Decreased muscle tone palpable following massage.

_____ Progress toward goal of independent car transfers and community ambulation 80%.

_____ Pt. squats with narrow base of support and rounded low back, placing object in front of knees.

*Thera-Band Resistive Exerciser, The Hygenic Corporation, Akron, Ohio.

Rewrite the following progress note so that the information is in the correct (i.e., logical) sequence. Then use the Guidelines for Critiquing the Progress Note (see p 142) and list how this note could be better written.

3-26-89

Pt. has met his STG of independent crutch walking. Says he needs to be able to climb three flights of stairs to get to his apartment. Will work on stair climbing next session. Handrail on L going up. Pt. crutch walked NWB, 300 ft on grass outside c̄ no assistance. R foot edema. Circumference equal L foot measurements. R knee flexion 10–110°. Pt. showing good progress in LE mobility. —Jim Jones, PTA

This note could be better written if:

Critique each of the following progress notes. They all relate to the same diagnosis and physical therapy problem.

Dx: 1 month post R ankle sprain

Pr: Limited R ankle ROM & strength interfering with ability to walk uphill to get to his house.

Progress Note 1:   4-20-95

S: Pt. states he's feeling better.

O: Gave US. Instructed in home ex. program. Instructed in amb. with cane.

A: Pt. tolerated tx well. Making progress.

P: Continue tx.—S. Student, SPTA/Wary T. Sign, PT

Progress Note 2: 4-20-95

S: Pt. reports less pain when walking but continues to have difficulty walking uphill.

O: Gave US to ankle, 1.5 w/cm², 5 min to prepare for stretching. Did contract–relax stretching exercises, dorsiflexion 0–5°, plantar flexion 0–40° (i.e., dorsiflex −5°, plantarflex 5–35°). Pt. correctly performed home ex. program using red Thera-Band to strengthen dorsiflexors, toe rises for plantarflexors and prolonged (30-min) stretch. See copy in chart. Pt. ambulated 100 ft, SEC, supervision for verbal cuing to minimize limp.

A: US & ex. effective in increasing ankle ROM. Pt. making progress toward goal of ① amb.

P: Continue per PT plan.—Better Student, SPTA/Will Sign, PTA

Progress Note 3: 4-20-95

S: Pt. states it is easier to walk. Reports increased pain when walking uphill.

O: Immersion US/R deltoid ligament, peroneus longus/brevis tendons/vigorous heat (1.5 w/cm²)/5 min/for stretching. Pain before tx 5/10, after tx 3/10. Contract–relax stretching for ankle ROM.

	4-15-95	4-20-95
Dorsiflexion	−5°	0–5°
Plantarflexion	5–35°	0–40°

Pt. correctly demonstrated home ex. program to strengthen all ankle muscles for stability using 3 sets of 10 reps with red therapeutic band & prolonged (30-min) stretch positions to increase ROM. See copy in chart. Pt. ambulated with SEC, mild-steppage gait, with slight foot slap at initial contact. Quality of gait improved with verbal cues to decrease knee flexion and use the ankle ROM. Ambulated on level sidewalk and level, uneven grass. _____

A: Pt.'s progress toward goal of Ⓘ amb. in community with amb. aid = 80%. US & ex. effective in increasing ankle ROM and quality of gait. _____

P: Continue per PT initial plan.—Good Student, SPTA/Will Sign, PT

_____

_____

_____

_____

_____

Progress Note 4: 4-20-95

Pt. describes a "stiffness" pain today following tx rated 3/10 vs. 5/10 before tx. States has difficulty walking uphill. PROM, 1 rep to assess all R ankle motions gives firm end feel. Slight softening of end feel after immersion US/1 MHz/vigorous heat (1.5 w/cm^2)/5 min/R deltoid ligament & peroneous longus & brevis tendons/pt. sitting/to increase elasticity, warm tissue to prepare for stretching. Contact–relax stretching, 3 reps each dorsiflexion & plantarflexion. _____

	4-15-95	4-20-95
Dorsiflexion	−5°	0–5°
Plantarflexion	5–35°	0–40°

Pt. correctly demonstrated dorsiflexion & plantarflexion strengthening exercises using red TheraBand, 3 sets of 10 reps, & 30-min prolonged stretch positions to increase ankle mobility per instructions in written home program. See copy in chart. Able to use blue TheraBand 10 reps. Pt. ambulated one city block on level sidewalk & level, uneven grass surface, using single-end cane, with supervision for verbal cuing to decrease knee flexion and use ankle dorsiflexion during initial swing. Quality of gait pattern improved by last 100 ft of the walk. Continues to demonstrate shortened stance phase, mild antalgic gait. Pt. has been seen 4×. 90% progress toward goal of Ⓘcommunity ambulation with or without ambulation aid. Ankle ROM increasing and strength gains with progression to more resistance (blue TheraBand). To be seen 4-25-95 & 4-30-95 (anticipated d/c session). Will add walking uphill next session. Will notify PT of possible d/c evaluation on 4-30-95.—Best Student, SPTA/Super Therapist, PTA, Lic. #123

_____

_____

_____

_____

_____

Use the Guidelines for Critiquing the Progress Note (see p 142) and critique the progress note in Figure 10–2.

_____

_____

_____

_____

_____

_____

_____

_____

_____

Rewrite and improve the progress notes in Chapter 4, Practice Exercises 3 and 5.

_____

_____

_____

_____

_____

_____

_____

_____

Below is a physical therapy initial evaluation. The exercises that follow relate to the information provided in this evaluation.

HOME HEALTH PHYSICAL THERAPY EVALUATION

Patient's name: _____ Mr. X _____ Physician: _____

Dx: Failed R hip prosthesis, R total hip revision.

History: 71 YO man who underwent R total hip revision and hospitalization 7-5-95 to 7-11-95. Pt. stated on first night home that he dropped R leg too far over side of bed and experienced a "pop." Currently experiences more side effects from this episode, denies increased pain on weight bearing but reports pain with spasms in R hip/thigh. Is up at night with frequent urination. States he previously could walk independently without an ambulation device, did his yardwork, and could drive. Has follow-up visit with Dr. in 2 weeks. He is retired and lives with his wife who states she is willing and able to assist him.

Physical Status: Communication—Pt. wears hearing aids, is difficult to understand due to decreased articulation, is oriented, has good attention span, has no memory deficits, is cooperative but presents with a flat affect. Palpation—Staples still in place in R hip incision, no derangement in hip noted. ROM—WFL in all joints except R hip flexion limited to 90° per total hip protocol and R hip abduction limited 25%. Moderate heel cord tightness noted. MMT—R hip abduction 2−/5, flexion 3−/5, requires assist for R SLR, R knee flexion/extension 3−/5, otherwise all WFL. Sitting balance good, standing balance fair and requires support of crutches, no problems with coordination.

Functional Status: ADLs—Ⓘ for feeding and hygiene/grooming, uses crutches, high chairs, and elevated toilet seat, needs assist for RLE when getting in/out of bed, taking a sponge bath, dressing lower extremities. Pt. ambulates with crutches and supervision limited distances within his home using a weight-bearing-as-tolerated pattern for R but does not bear wt. on heel. Physical environment—House with several steps to enter, low-pile carpet or tile throughout, single bed with bathroom down the hall.

Physical Therapy Problem:
1. Decreased strength/ROM RLE interfering with transfer ability from bed and chairs. Dependent sit ↔ supine and bed mobility.

2. Limited crutch ambulation within home secondary to decreased RLE strength and endurance.

Functional Outcomes:
1. Safe and Ⓘ transfers from variety of surfaces in home in 3 weeks.

2. Safe and Ⓘ household ambulation with appropriate ambulation device for 5 or more min, up/down stairs to exit home in 3 weeks.

3. Wife/pt. to carry out home exercise program correctly and Ⓘ in 1 week.

Treatment Plan:
1. Home program of ROM and strengthening exercises to increase ROM and strength of RLE to allow safe and Ⓘ transfers.

2. Structured home ambulation program to increase ambulation endurance to 5 min and to improve safety.

3. Gait training on stairs to allow exit from home.

4. Transfer training from a variety of surfaces with emphasis on getting in/out of bed.

Treatment will be 2×/week for 3 weeks. Rehab potential good for meeting goals in 3 weeks and discharge. Plan was reviewed with patient and wife with patient agreeable.

Initial Treatment:

7-12-95   Gait training and transfer training in/out of bed initiated. Pt. ambulated touching R toes only on initial contact. Able to lightly place heel on floor with verbal cues. Pt. required frequent cuing for heel/toe pattern. In/out bed transfers required moderate assist with LEs. Reviewed total hip protocol with pt. and wife; they seemed to understand. Pt. correctly demonstrated home exercises after instructions (see copy in chart), and wife was able to assist pt. with R hip abduction and SLR. Will refer pt. to Joe Jones, PTA, for next 5 visits, and PT will see pt. on 6th visit. Anticipate discharge evaluation at that time. **Signed:** Mary Williams, MS, PT, Lic. #123

EXERCISES

7.1. You are Joe Jones, PTA, and you have just made a home visit and treated Mr. X. Review the following notes you took during the treatment session, and write your progress note.

7-17-95

Pt. in good mood, no c/o pain.

Exercises: 10 reps each. Standing at kitchen counter—toe raises, partial knee bends, hip abd, gentle hyperextension, hamstring curls. Supine—SLR with approx. 60–70% assist, bent knee abd.

Sitting—long arc quads.

Amb. in house, good, supervision, 3 point, step-through gait, 1 crutch on L, erect posture, heel/toe pattern. Ⓘ up/down stairs in house and porch.

Said able to shower with SBA from wife. Used high stool, sit, swing leg over tub, stand. C/o intense mm spasms after sitting in easy chair. C/o "clink" in hip area with active extension.

Recommend raising chair on platform, notify Dr if spasms persist/worse, perform extension ex. gently and stop if feels clink again, recommend use 2 crutches if fatigued.

Next visit = 7-25-95.

_____

_____

_____

_____

_____

_____

7.2. Use the Guidelines for Critiquing the Progress Note (see p 142) and identify ways to improve the following progress note:

7-25-95   **Pr:** Decreased ROM & strength RLE interfering with transfers & ambulation safety and endurance.

_____

S: "I saw the doctor yesterday. He thinks everything looks good."

O: Pt. c/o pain when walking outside. Ambulated pt. with one crutch, 3 point heel/toe gait pattern. Instructed on stairs. Pt. states he is bearing about 75% of his wt. on RLE. RLE exercises 10×. Instructed pt. to hold abduction for 3 counts to increase difficulty.

A: Pt. pleased with progress. Progress toward goals 95%. Needs two more visits.

P: Will notify PT about discharge evaluation next week.—Joe Jones, PTA

_____

_____

_____

_____

7.3. Critique the following progress note:

7-27-95   **Pr:** Decreased ROM and strength RLE interfering with transfers and ambulation safety and endurance.

_____

Pt. described discomfort in R hip when leg tires as "hip socket feels thicker." While ambulating with cane during treatment session, pt. reported he didn't feel as steady as with the crutch and the cane is harder on his L wrist. States he continues to have his wife stand by when he is showering. Pt. Ⓘ performed his THA exercises supine in bed 10 reps each/heel slides, abduction with powder board, SLR, short arc quads over folded pillow, ankle pumps, isometrics for quads, gluts, hams/RLE exercises standing at kitchen counter per previous note with encouragement to hold abduction 3 counts/reminders to breathe during the exercise. Pt. demonstrated Ⓘ bed mobility and sit ⟷ stand from elevated easy chair/elevated toilet seat/kitchen chair/bed. Pt. Ⓘ ambulated outside 4 min with one crutch, heel/toe, step through, full wt. bearing gait, demonstrating good balance and erect posture. Ⓘ went up/down 3 stairs, no railing. Pt. ambulated with single-end cane in house for first time with min. assist for sense of security and verbal cues, demonstrating slight trunk lean to R (Trendelenburg lurch). Pt./wife encouraged to practice walking short distances in the house with the cane. Progress toward functional outcomes listed in initial eval.: #1 met; #2 80%, needs to build endurance to 5-min walk and gain confidence with cane; #3 met. Pt. needs one more visit to work on ambulation and balance with cane and anticipate discharge at that time. Will schedule PT for discharge evaluation.

—Joe Jones, PTA, Lic. #123

_____

_____

_____

_____

7.4. Refer to the initial evaluation for Mr. X with the failed hip prosthesis. The following questions relate to this evaluation.

a. Read the physical therapy problems identified in the evaluation. List the impairments and the functional limitations.

_____

_____

b. Copy the functional outcomes planned in the evaluation. *Circle* the action, *underline* how the outcome will be measured, and *draw a line through* the time period.

_____

_____

_____

c. Copy the treatment plans from the evaluation. *Circle* the treatment, *underline* how the plan will be measured, and *draw a line through* the frequency and duration. Describe how the impairments will be treated and describe the functional activities.

_____

_____

_____

d. Critique the progress note you wrote in Exercise 7.1. (p 153).

_____

_____

_____

_____

Below is a physical therapy initial evaluation. The series of questions that follows relates to the information provided in this evaluation.

LONG-TERM CARE FACILITY: PHYSICAL THERAPY EVALUATION

Patient's name: _____   Date of initial evaluation: 8-7-94

Room number: _____   Physician: _____

Date of birth:

Diagnosis: Dementia, peripheral vascular disease, atrial fibrillation, heel pressure ulcers bilaterally.

Onset: 7-31-94.

Patient evaluated at bedside. Nursing reported they do two-person lifts to move patient in bed and to transfer to chair. Patient alert but communicated in a confused manner. Pressure ulcers observed on both heels, L greater than R. R wound bed covered with black, thick eschar. Borders detached with red granulation tissue. Significant callous formation around perimeter. No foul odor, minimal drainage. L wound red around edge, significant callous formation around edge. Wound bed covered with blister with dark purple discoloration. Open area in blister/broken blister with minimal drainage, no foul odor.

	R Heel	**L Heel**
Stage:	Stage III	Stage II
Shape:	Round	Round
Size:	3.9 (horiz) × 3.4 (vert) cm	Open area 4.3 × 7.2 cm
		Blistered area 6 × 7.3 cm
		Red periphery 11 × 12 cm
Drainage:	Minimum, serous	Minimum, serous

Physical Therapy Problem: Bil. heel pressure ulcers with necrotic tissue and blister interfering with healing, bed mobility, and transfers.

Goals: Debride necrotic tissue in 3 days for clean wound with healthy tissue to enhance healing for eventual assisted bed mobility and assisted pivot transfers.

Treatment Plan: Pulsavac* jet lavage to clean wound and loosen blister and necrotic tissue, followed by debridement of loose skin and necrotic tissue to promote healing, both heels, 1×/day for 3 days.

Initial Treatment: Standard Pulsavac treatment/both heels/bedside/sterile towel under feet with pad underneath. Loose skin from blister debrided on L, healthy tissue under. Eschar trimmed from edges on R. Feet wrapped in sterile towel following, nursing notified; they will dress wounds.—PT signature, Lic. #xxxxxx

Instructions
Answer the following questions that refer to the initial evaluation of the patient with bilateral pressure ulcers on heels.

1. Does the evaluation contain subjective data? Explain.

_____

_____

_____

2. Does the objective data paint a picture of the wounds? Explain.

_____

_____

_____

3. Is the objective data reproducible? Explain.

_____

_____

_____

---

*Pulsavac III Wound Debridement System, Zimmer Patient Care Division, Dover, OH.

4. What is the impairment?

_____

_____

_____

5. What is the functional limitation?

_____

_____

_____

6. What is the purpose of the treatment?

_____

_____

_____

7. What is the frequency and duration of the treatment plan?

_____

_____

_____

8. Copy the goal. *Circle* the action, *underline* the criteria for the goal to be met, and *draw a line through* the time period.

_____

_____

_____

9. Assume you are an experienced PTA and have had extra training in wound care. The PT has confidence in your skills to debride and treat these wounds.

a. Can you duplicate the treatment? Explain.

_____

_____

_____

b. How will you know when to have the PT do the discharge evaluation?

_____

_____

_____

c. List ways you can document the progress.

_____

_____

_____

Many topics about producing quality documentation have been presented in this text. Go back to Chapter 1 and reread the story about the PT's court experience in 1968. Many of the topics in the text are illustrated or suggested in the story. List as many topics as you can.

_____

_____

_____

_____

Bibliography

American Physical Therapy Association and the Section on Pediatrics: Individualized educational program and individualized family service plan. In Martin, KD (ed.): Physical Therapy Practice in Educational Environments: Policies and Guidelines. APTA, Alexandria, VA, 1990, p 6.1.

Anderson, K, and Anderson, L: Mosby's Pocket Dictionary of Medicine, Nursing, & Allied Health. CV Mosby, St. Louis, 1990.

Bernstein, F, et al: Insurance reimbursement and the physical therapist: Documentation for outpatient physical therapy; Guidelines based on California state law. Clin Manage Phys Ther 2:28–33, 1987.

Brown, SR: Physical therapy documentation—Part III. The Pyramid 17:2, 1987.

Cutone, J: One PTA's experience: Team collaboration in the school setting. PT Magazine 3:48, 1994.

Davis, C, and Lippert, L: Facilitators: Reaching agreement about key content areas in PTA curricula. PTA educators colloquium, September 16–17, 1994, Minneapolis. Proceedings to be published by American Physical Therapy Association, Alexandria, VA.

Delitto, A, and Snyder-Mackler, L: The diagnostic process. Examples in orthopedic physical therapy. Phys Ther 3:203, 1995.

Duncan, P: Balance Dysfunction and Motor Control Theory. Workshop notes, April 7–8, 1995, College of St. Scholastica, Duluth, MN.

Esposto, L: Applying functional outcome assessment to Medicare documentation. In Stewart, DL, and Abeln, SH (eds): Documenting Functional Outcomes in Physical Therapy. Mosby–Year Book, St. Louis, 1993.

Feitelberg, SB (Presenter): A systematic approach to documentation: The basis for successful reimbursement. American Rehabilitation Educational Network (AREN) teleconference, March 19, 1991.

Government Affairs Department: Physical therapy practice without referral: "Direct access." American Physical Therapy Association, Alexandria, VA, 1992.

Guccione, A: Functional assessment. In O'Sullivan, SB, and Schmitz, JJ (eds): Physical Rehabilitation, Assessment, and Treatment. FA Davis, Philadelphia, 1994.

Hebert, L.: Basics of Medicare documentation for physical therapy. Clinical Management, 1:3, 1981, p 13.

Hill, JR: The Problem-Oriented Approach to Physical Therapy Care. American Physical Therapy Association, Alexandria, VA, 1987.

Jette, AM: Using health-related quality of life measures in physical therapy outcomes research. Phys Ther 8:528, 1993.

Langley, GB, and Sheppeard, H. The visual analogue scale: Its use in pain measurement. Rheumatol Int 5:145, 1985.

Lunning, S (Presenter): Opportunity or chaos? Prepare for the future in physical therapy. Minnesota Chapter American Physical Therapy Association Peer Review Workshop, May 10, 1994, Virginia, MN.

Lupi-Williams, FA: The PTA role & function: An analysis in three parts. Part 1: Education. Clin Manage Phys Ther 3:3, 1983.

McGuire, DB: The measurement of clinical pain. Nurs Res 3:152, 1984.

Melzack, R: The McGill Pain Questionnaire: Major properties and scoring methods. Pain 1:277, 1975.

Moffat, M: Foreward. Journal of Physical Therapy Education 9:35, Fall 1995.

Montgomery, P, and Connolly, B: Motor Control and Physical Therapy: Theoretical Framework, Practical Application, First Edition. Chattanooga Group, Hixson, TN, 1991.

Nagi, SZ: Disability and rehabilitation. Ohio State University Press, Columbus, 1969.

Ransford, A, et al: The pain drawing as an aid to the psychologic evaluation of patients with low-back pain. Spine 1:127, 1976.

Rogers, J: PTA utilization: The big picture. Clin Manage Phys Ther 11:4, July/August 1991, p 8.

Rose, S: Diagnosis: Defining the term. Phys Ther 69:162, 1989.

Stewart, DL, and Abeln, SH: Documenting Functional Outcomes in Physical Therapy. Mosby–Year Book, St. Louis, 1993.

Swanson, G: Essentials for the Future of Physical Therapy, Every Therapist's Concern. A Continuing Education Course. Minnesota Chapter American Physical Therapy Association, December 1995, Duluth, MN.

Task Force on Standards for Measurement in Physical Therapy: Standards for tests and measurements in physical therapy practice. Phys Ther 71:589, 1991.

Terminology Task Force of the Acute Care/Hospital Clinical Practice Section of American Physical Therapy Association: Common Terminology, First Draft. Decatur, GA, November 1994.

Thomas, CL (ed): Taber's Cyclopedic Medical Dictionary, Seventeenth Edition. FA Davis, Philadelphia, 1993.

Yaeger, J: Effective listening techniques. Notes from Mgt 503, Oral Communication. Masters in Management Program. College of St. Scholastica, Duluth, MN, 1990.

Glossary

Accountable: Responsible, capable of explaining oneself.

Accredit: To supply with credentials or authority.

Accreditation: Granting of approval to an institution by an official review board after the institution has met specific requirements.

Adhesive capsulitis: A condition characterized by adhesions and shortening or tightening of the connective tissue sleeve that encases a joint.

Ambulate: To walk about.

American Physical Therapy Association: Professional organization representing the physical therapy profession, the occupation consisting of professionals and technicians trained to provide the medical rehabilitative service of physical therapy.

Antalgic: Painful or indicating the presence of pain.

Anterior capsule: Front portion of the joint connective tissue sleeve.

Assessment: Measurement, quantification, or placement of a value or label on something; assessment is often confused with evaluation; an assessment results from the act of assessing.*

Ataxia: Condition characterized by impaired ability to coordinate movement. Ataxic gait is a staggering, uncoordinated walk.

Audit: Examination of records to check accuracy and compliance with professional standards.

Authenticate: To verify, to prove, to establish as worthy of belief.

Autonomy: Independence, ability to self-govern.

Biomechanics: Study of mechanical laws and their application to living organisms, especially the human body.

Circumduct: To move the joint in a circular manner.

Clinical decision: Determination that relates to direct patient care, indirect patient care, acceptance of patients for treatment, and whether patients should be referred to other practitioners.† A diagnosis that leads a therapist to take an action is a form of a clinical decision; clinical decisions result in actions; when direct supporting evidence for clinical decisions is lacking, such decisions are based on clinical opinions.

Collaborate: To work together, to cooperate.

Concentric contraction: Muscle contraction that moves the muscle from a resting, lengthened position to a shortened position; a muscle contraction in which the insertion and origin move closer together.

Continuum: A continuous extent, succession, or whole.

Coordination: Muscle action of the appropriate intensity, timing, and sequencing to produce a smooth, controlled, purposeful movement.

Criteria: Requirements, standards, rules.

Data: Information, especially information organized for analysis or used as the basis for a decision.

Direct access: Legislation that enables the consumer to enter the medical care system by going directly to a PT. The patient needing physical therapy treatment does not need to be referred to a PT by a physician.

Discharge evaluation: Made only by a PT on termination of treatment by the PT. It contains recommendations and decisions about future treatment.

Discharge summary: A document that may be written by the PTA stating the treatments provided and the status of the patient at time of discharge. If this document contains recommendations or decisions about future treatment, it is considered an evaluation and must be written by the PT.

Documentation: Written information supplying proof, a written record, supporting references.

Duration: Period of time in which something persists or exists.

Eccentric contraction: A muscle contraction that moves the muscle from a shortened position to its lengthened or resting position; muscle contraction in which the insertion and origin move away from each other.

Edema: Swelling; accumulation of fluid in the tissues.

Efficacy: Effectiveness, ability to achieve results.

Evaluation: Judgment based on a measurement; often confused with assessment and examination; evaluations are judgments of the value or worth of something.*

Examination: Test or a group of tests used for the purpose of obtaining measurements or data.*

Extension: Movement of a joint in which the angle between the two adjoining bones increases.

Facilitate: To enhance or help an action or function.

Femur: Thigh bone.

Flexion: Movement of a joint in which the angle between the two adjoining bones decreases.

Fractured: Broken. Typically refers to broken bones.

Frequency: Number of times something occurs, number of repetitions, number of treatment sessions.

Gait: Walking pattern.

Girth: Distance around something, circumference.

Goniometry: Procedure for measuring the range of motion angles of a joint.

Hamstrings: Common name for the group of three muscles located on the posterior thigh.

Hip extensors: Common name for the group of muscles that produce extension motion of the hip joint.

Hypertonus: Excessive muscle tone or prolonged muscle contraction.

Incident: Distinct occurrence; an event inconsistent with usual routine or treatment procedure; an accident.

Incident report: Documentation required when an unusual event occurs in a clinic or medical facility.

Individual educational program: Written statement outlining the goals and objectives for the services provided to meet a physically disabled child's educational needs.

Informed consent: Permission or agreement for medical treatment based on knowledge of all the information about the treatment.

Initial and mid swing: Portions of the walking pattern when the heel and then the toes leave the ground and the leg swings to the point where the hip is at 0° flexion or extension.

Internship: Period of time during which a medical professional in training provides clinical care under supervision.

Joint Commission on Accreditation of Healthcare Organizations: Agency with the responsibility to ensure that hospitals and medical centers follow federal and state regulations and meet the standards necessary for the provision of safe and appropriate health care.

Laceration: Torn, jagged wound.

Lag: To fall behind, not keep up, develop slowly, weaken, or slacken.

Lower extremity: Area that includes the thigh, lower leg, and foot.

Medicaid: Federally funded, state-administered health insurance for eligible individuals with low income who are too young to qualify for Medicare.

Medical diagnosis: Identification of a systemic disease or disorder based on the findings from a physician's examination and diagnostic test.

Medicare: Federally funded national health insurance for certain persons older than 65.

Mobilization techniques: Manual techniques or procedures used by physical therapy professionals to increase the range of motion of a joint.

Modality: Method of therapy or treatment procedure.

Muscle spasms: Persistent, involuntary contractions of a muscle or certain groups of muscle fibers within the muscle.

Negligence: State of being extremely careless or lacking in concern.

Neuromusculoskeletal: Pertaining to the nervous system, the muscular system, and the skeletal system.

Occupational therapist: Trained health care professional who provides occupational therapy.

Occupational therapy assistant: Trained health care technician who provides occupational therapy under the supervision of an occupational therapist.

Orthopedics: Branch of medicine devoted to the study and treatment of the skeletal system and its joints, muscles, and associated structures.

Palpable: Able to be felt or touched.

Parameters: Limits or boundaries; a value or constant used to describe or measure a set of data representing a physiologic function or system.

Paraparesis: Partial paralysis or extreme weakness.

Pathokinesiologic: Pertaining to the study of movements relating to a given disorder.

Pathologic: Pertaining to a condition that is caused by or involves a disease.

Pathology: Study of the characteristics, causes, and effects of disease.

Physical therapy: The treatment of impairments and functional limitations by physical means such as exercise, education and training, heat, light, electricity, water, cold, ultrasound, massage, and manual therapy to improve or restore the patient's ability to function in his or her environment. Physical therapy is provided by trained persons who have graduated from accredited physical therapy and physical therapist assistant schools.

Physical Therapy Practice Act: Legislation in each state that defines and regulates the practice or provision of physical therapy services.

Physical therapy problem: Identification of the neuromusculoskeletal dysfunction and resulting functional limitation that is treatable by physical therapy.

Physician assistants: Trained technicians performing medical care under the supervision of a physician.

Problem-oriented: Based on or directed toward the problem, as in the medical record organized around the identification of the medical problems.

Prone: Horizontal and face-down position.

Psoriasis: A common, chronic, inheritable skin disorder characterized by circumscribed red patches covered by thick, dry, silvery, adherent scales.

Quadriparesis: Partial paralysis or extreme weakness of arms, legs, and trunk resulting from injury to spinal nerves in the cervical spine.

Quality assurance: Title of the department, usually in health care facilities, that reviews medical charts to identify when regulations and standards are not being met or when unsafe or inappropriate medical care is provided.

Quality assurance committee: Group that performs chart reviews.

Rehabilitation facilities: Clinics or institutions that provide rehabilitation services such as physical therapy, occupational therapy, speech pathology, psychological services, social services, orthotics and prosthetics, and patient and family education.

Reimbursement: Payment for services.

Release of information form: Document that the patient signs to give permission for the person(s) named in the document to receive information about the patient's medical condition and treatment.

Reliable: Dependable, reproducible.

Retrospective: Looking back on, contemplating, or directed to the past.

Rule of confidentiality: A principle that information about patients should not be revealed to anyone not authorized to receive the information.

Signs: Characteristics or indications of disease or dysfunction determined by objective tests, measurements, or observations.

Source-oriented: Organized around the source of the information, as in the medical record organized according to the various disciplines providing and documenting the care.

Speech pathologist: Trained professional who diagnoses and treats abnormalities of speech.

Status quo: No change in a specified state or condition.

Symptoms: Subjective characteristics or indications of disease or dysfunction as perceived by the patient.

Systemic: Pertaining to the whole body.

Tactile: Pertaining to the sense of touch.

Vital signs: Measurements of pulse rate, respiration rate, body temperature, and blood pressure.

Workers' compensation: State- and business-funded health insurance that manages and funds medical care for persons injured on the job.

---

*Task Force on Standards for Measurement in Physical Therapy: Standards for tests and measurement in physical therapy practice. Phys Ther 71:589, 1991.

†This definition is modified from that presented by Charles Magistro at a conference on Clinical Decision Making held under APTA auspices in October 1988 in Lake of the Ozarks, MO.

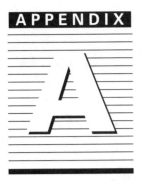
Abbreviations

↑ increase

↓ decrease

// parallel

1× one time, one person

2° secondary to

ā before

abd/add abduction/adduction

ADL activities of daily living

AFO ankle foot orthosis

amb. ambulation

appts appointments

APTA American Physical Therapy Association

AAROM active assistive range of motion

AROM active range of motion

assist assistance

B bilateral, both

bid twice a day

bil. bilateral

BLE both lower extremities

BPM beats per minute

c̄ with

CARF Commission on Accreditation of Rehabilitation Facilities

CCs chief complaints

c/o complains of, complaint(s) of

CP compression pump

CPM continuous passive motion machine

CVA cerebral vascular accident

d/c discharged, discontinued

DEP data, evaluation, performance goals

DJD degenerative joint disease

DOB date of birth

Dx diagnosis

ER emergency room, external rotation

ex. exercise

F female

FAROM functional active range of motion

FES functional electrical stimulation

flex flexion

FOR functional outcome report

F/U follow up

FWW, fw/w front wheeled walker

Fx fracture(d)

gastrocs gastrocnemius muscles

gluts gluteals

GMT gross muscle test

Gt. gait

hams hamstrings

HNP herniated nucleus pulposus

Hx history

Ⓘ independent(ly)

ICP intermittent compression pump

IEP individual education program

int. internal

JCAHO Joint Commission on Accreditation of Healthcare Organizations

L left

L5 5th lumbar vertebra

lat. lateral

LBP low back pain

LLE left lower extremity

LOB loss of balance

LUE left upper extremity

M male

MH moist heat

min. minimal, minimum

mmHg millimeters of mercury

mm(s) muscle(s)

MMT manual muscle test

N/A not applicable

neg. negative

noc. night
NWB non–weight-bearing
OOB out of bed
OP outpatient
OT occupational therapist
p̄ after
P poor muscle grade strength
per by
PM afternoon
POMR problem-oriented medical record
PRE progressive resistive exercise
PRN as needed
PROM passive range of motion
PSP problem, status, plan
PSPG problem, status, plan, goals
pt. patient
PT physical therapist
PTA physical therapist assistant
PWB partial weight bearing
quads quadriceps
R right
RA rheumatoid arthritis
re: regarding
reps repetitions
ret. return
RLE right lower extremity
r/o rule out
ROM range of motion
rot. rotation
RUE right upper extremity
SBA standby assist

SCI spinal cord injury
SEC single-end cane
SLR straight leg raise
SOMR source-oriented medical record
STG short-term goal
str. strength
strep *Streptococcus*
SWD shortwave diathermy
Sx symptoms
TDD tentative discharge data
TDP tentative discharge plan
temp. temperature
THA total hip arthroplasty
ther. ex. therapeutic exercise
tid three times a day
TKA total knee arthroplasty
TKE terminal knee extension
TMJ temporomandibular joint
trng. training
TWB touch weight bearing
tx treatment
UE upper extremity
UED1 upper extremity diagonal 1
w/ with
WC, w/c wheelchair
WFL within functional limits
w/o without
WNL within normal limits
wt. weight
YO year(s) old

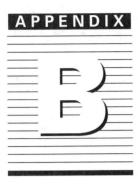

Documenting Modality Treatments

It is not easy for one to document treatment procedures thoroughly enough so that the treatment can be reproduced by another PTA or PT and still keep the progress note as brief as possible. The following is a method for providing the appropriate information in a short format.

SUGGESTED MODALITY DOCUMENTATION STYLE

In the modality documentation style, the information is placed in a continuous line separated by slashes. A list of information that should be included for the treatment to be reproducible is provided on page 82. The information is documented as illustrated here but does not have to be placed in this order. Type of modality/dosage or intensity/treatment area/time/patient position/frequency/purpose.

Examples

Direct contact US/3 MHz/mild heat at 0.5 w/cm²/right TMJ/sitting/5 min/to decrease inflammation.

Direct contact US/1 MHz/moderate heat/7 min/left middle trapezius & rhomboid/prone/to relax spasm.

Direct contact US/1 MHz/vigorous heat/5 min/L shoulder, anterior capsule/sitting/to prepare for stretching.

Induction SWD/large pad/dose III/vigorous heat/L1 to S2/prone/20 min to prepare for stretching.

Intermittent cervical traction/Saunders halter/supine/15 lb/30 sec on, 10 sec off/20 min/to stretch C1–C4 cervical extensors.

Immersion US/1 MHz/right deltoid ligament/sitting/vigorous heat at 2 w/cm²/10 min/to prepare for stretching

Static pelvic traction/L4–L5/prone/100 lb/10 min max. or until pain centralizes/to reduce disc bulge.

Ice massage/standard procedure/to numbing response/R wrist extensors' tendons at origin/sitting, shoulder abducted 90°, elbow flexed 90° on pillow/after exercise/to minimize inflammatory response.

Hot packs/R biceps femoris muscle belly/moderate heat/prone/20 min/to increase circulation for healing.

Foot whirlpool/110°/decubitus on L lateral malleolus/sitting in wheelchair/for mechanical debridement/20 min.

ICP/50 lb/30 sec on, 10 sec off/RUE/elevated 45°/supine/3 hr/to decrease edema.

FES/L anterior tibialis/monopolar/one channel, three leads/two 2-inch square electrodes/origin & insertion/nontreatment electrode under R thigh/30 pps/15 min/motor response/pt. semi-sitting/for muscle re-education and AAROM.

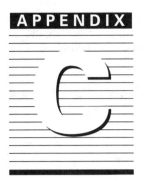

Dictation Guidelines

In some clinical facilities you will dictate your progress notes instead of writing them. You will dictate or speak into a recording device (such as a small tape recorder or into a telephone), and a medical transcriber will listen to the tape and type your note. The typed note will be returned to you for proofreading and your signature. When you are first learning to dictate progress notes, take the time to write the note first on scrap paper, and then you can read it out loud into the recorder. After you become accustomed to the dictation procedure, you will be able to compose the note and dictate it simultaneously.

GUIDELINES FOR CLEAR DICTATION

1. Each facility will have guidelines for you. In one clinic, the transcriber may be so skilled in typing physical therapy documentation that you will do little more than dictate the content. Another clinic may require that you give instructions to the transcriber and dictate punctuation.

2. Use proper sentence structure and punctuation, although you can eliminate some wording to keep the note brief.

3. Introduce your dictation by telling the transcriber *who you are,* that this is a *progress note,* the *name of your patient,* and the *date of treatment.*

4. Spell out any foreign or unusual names of muscles, treatment techniques, or diagnoses. Clarify *ab*duct and *add*uct by spelling out the word.

5. Tell the transcriber when you are starting or finishing a note on a particular patient or date, particularly if you are dictating more than one note on a tape.

6. Stating "operator" just before your instructions alerts the transcriber that *instructions* are to follow, not content.

7. Tell the transcriber what letters you want capitalized. However, you can assume the transcriber will automatically capitalize the first letter of each sentence.

    Example: You might say, "Patient's (operator: all in caps) ROM (operator: end of caps) is 0–90 degrees for left knee flexion."

8. Tell the transcriber when you are moving to a new heading.

    Example: "(operator: new heading, all in caps) objective" will come back to you typed "OBJECTIVE."

9. You may need to dictate some of the punctuation.

Example: You want your note to read, "<u>Transfers:</u> Ⓘ out recliner, on/off toilet, bed after four tries" Your dictation should sound like this: "(Operator: underline capital T) transfers colon independent out recliner comma on slash off toilet comma bed after four tries period."

10. Give your full legal name with your proper abbreviated title (SPTA or PTA) at the end of the dictation.

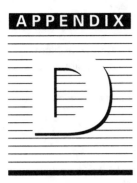

Answers to Review Exercises

CHAPTER 1 Review exercises are on page 11.

1. If there is no documentation that medical care was provided, then it is assumed the care did not occur or was not given.

2. First, physicians prescribed the therapy and told the PT exactly what treatments to do. Later, the prescription just referred the patient to the PT with a diagnosis, and the PT could evaluate and decide what treatments were appropriate. Finally, direct access legislation allows the PT to see a patient, evaluate, and treat without the patient first going to a physician for referral.

3. First, the PT was a technician, following the exact orders of the physician. Later, the PT added evaluation skills and decision-making as to treatment plans, and the PTA carried out the plans under PT supervision. Now the PT consults, evaluates, and recognizes when to refer a patient to a physician or another more appropriate health care provider. The PTA continues to carry out the treatment plan, but does not require on-site supervision and is part of the PT–PTA team.

4. Direct access means a person can see a PT without obtaining a physician's referral. The first medical professional seeing the patient may be a PT, and the PT may refer the patient to another appropriate health care provider. Thus a person can access the health care system through physical therapy.

5. The costs of providing health care.

6. The medical record is (1) a record of the quality of the medical care provided to the patient, (2) a legal document providing evidence of the care, and (3) the method by which third-party payers determine the value of the care provided and reimbursement for that care.

7. The record is audited to ensure that the standards and criteria for quality care and documentation are followed.

8. The federal government, state government, accrediting agencies, professional agencies, and the individual health facility.

9. Following the policies and procedures where you work ensures that your documentation will meet the necessary standards or criteria.

CHAPTER 2 Review exercises are on page 21.

1. a. **Data:** The subjective and objective information that is gathered about the patient and why he or she is seeking medical treatment.

b. **Problems:** The problems that require medical treatment as determined by interpretation of the data.

c. **Treatment plan:** The description of the treatment appropriate for the problems.

d. **Purpose, goals, desired outcomes:** Statements describing what the treatment should accomplish.

e. **Treatment procedures administered:** A record of the treatments provided through progress notes, flow charts, checklists, or brief statements.

f. **Results or effectiveness of the treatment:** Statements as to whether or not the treatment accomplished its intended purpose or goal.

2. **Subjective data** constitute the information provided by the patient or a representative of the patient. These data are what the patient tells the medical person. **Objective data** constitute the information gathered by a health care provider through tests, measurements, observations, and examinations. This information can be reproduced by another health care provider with the same training.

3. **Symptoms** are the feelings, experiences, or complaints the patient describes that cause the patient to seek medical attention. The objective information gathered from tests, measurements, and observations are the **signs** of the disease or pathology.

4. The **medical diagnosis** is a systemic disease or disorder determined by the physician through physical examination and diagnostic tests. The **physical therapy problem** is the identification of a dysfunction of the neuromusculoskeletal system resulting in one or more functional limitations or difficulties causing the patient to seek physical therapy. The physical therapy problem can be the medical diagnosis, or a patient may have both a medical diagnosis and a PT problem.

5. The PT is responsible for writing all evaluations, goals or outcomes, and treatment plans for the patient. Both the PT and the PTA write progress notes.

6. The three types of evaluations are **initial, interim, and discharge.** The PTA may assist the PT with the evaluation by taking notes, performing and recording the results of tests or measurements within the scope of PTA practice, and establishing a rapport with the patient. The PTA plans the treatment sessions based on the PT's treatment plan, objectives, and goals or functional outcomes.

7. A **discharge evaluation** summarizes the treatment the patient received, discusses the results, identifies whether or not the treatment was effective, and makes recommendations or states what is planned for the patient after discharge. This evaluation must be documented by a PT. A PTA is permitted to write a **discharge summary** that simply lists the treatments provided and describes the patient's status at discharge time. In the discharge summary, the PTA is not to make recommendations or decisions on the basis of the information about the patient's treatment following discharge. The final note in the PT chart about the patient must be written by the PT.

CHAPTER 3   Review exercises are on page 41.

1. **SOMR** is the abbreviation for source-oriented medical record. The SOMR is organized into sections according to the disciplines or medical services providing the information. There is a physicians' information section, a nursing section, a physical therapy section, a laboratory test results section, and so on. **POMR** is the abbreviation for problem-oriented medical record. The POMR is organized into sections according to the information or documentation content, and the content focuses on the problems being treated. The sections consist of the data, problems, treatment plans, progress notes, and discharge notes. Each discipline writes its information in the appropriate section. For example, physical therapy notes and nursing notes would be together in the progress note section, addressing the problem being treated.

2. **S** stands for subjective, and this section contains information told to the therapist by the patient or someone representing the patient.

O stands for objective, and this section contains information gathered from tests, measurements, and observations that can be reproduced by someone else with the same training.

A stands for assessment, and this section contains statements that interpret the subjective and objective data. Treatment goals as well as treatment effectiveness and outcome are recorded here.

P stands for plan, and this section states the treatment plan or what will happen in the next treatment session.

3. **PSPG, DEP,** and **FOR** are other models for organizing evaluation and progress note content. PSPG stands for problem, status, plan, and goals. DEP stands for data, evaluation, and performance goals. FOR is the abbreviation for functional outcome report.

4. The PTA can adapt to any organization model by logically sequencing the progress note information in a problem-solving manner. First, identify the problem about which the note is written. Next, report the data gathered during treatment and interpret these data by showing how the information relates to the treatment objectives and functional goals established in the PT's initial evaluation. Finally, report what is planned for the next session. The PTA can easily organize this information into any format.

5. **Checklist, flow charts, fill-in-the-blank forms:** Typically used in hospitals, long-term care facilities, and rehabilitation centers.

   Narrative or outlined notes, dictated and typed or handwritten: Used in all facilities and can be combined with checklists, flow charts, and other forms.

   Letter: Commonly used by private practice facilities to communicate with the physician about the patient's treatment progress.

   Individualized educational program: Used in the schools when a physically disabled child requires specialized services such as physical therapy to assist in his or her education.

   Cardex: Some facilities keep up-to-date treatment plans on cards kept within the physical therapy department. These are used by the treating therapists for quick references and are not part of the patient's medical record.

   Medicare standardized forms: Documentation forms that health care personnel are required to use when treating patients who have Medicare insurance. These forms are common in long-term care facilities, rehabilitation centers, home health care agencies, and hospitals.

6. Using symbols to describe the patient's functional status, the PTA can complete the center section of the recertification form and provide the information to the PT. The PTA *should not complete* the form because it is intended to be an evaluation.

7. The PTA should always follow the facility's documentation policies, procedures, and format.

CHAPTER 4   Review exercises are on page 57.

1. The progress note is the record of the treatment procedures administered. It is written proof that the PT's treatment plan was carried out and is documentation of the effectiveness of the treatment. Both PTs and PTAs write progress notes, but the PTA's main documentation responsiblity is writing the progress note. Progress notes are written daily for acute care patients and weekly or less often for patients receiving treatment for chronic conditions. Frequency depends on the facility's procedures.

2. Progress notes can be written in SOAP outline; in paragraph style narration; in a combination of checklists, flow sheets, and narrative; on computer software forms; dictated and typed or handwritten; or in formats (e.g., DEP, FOR, PSPG) according to the facility's preference.

3. **Be accurate:** Information about the patient's medical care must be thorough and accurate in case it must be recalled later in court or if questions arise.

   Be brief: Notes must be relevant to the problem being treated and must be thorough, but they should be short so that they can be read quickly. Be concise and to the point; do not use excess words.

Be clear: Everyone who reads the note must be able to understand its meaning. Handwritten notes must be legible, and punctuation, grammar, and spelling must be correct.

Date and sign all entries: It must be clear when the note was written and who wrote it for reference later if questions arise.

Use black ink: You may also use a color of ink that will distinguish the original document from a copy. The document should be clear when photocopied.

Do not allow opportunity for the record to be changed or falsified: The note must be accurate, so you should not leave spaces where information could be inserted and should not use an erasable pen that would enable your information to be changed. Do not erase errors, but instead draw a line through the mistake and date and initial above it so that it is clear who made the change.

Documentation should be timely: The note will be more accurate if it is written as soon as possible after the patient's treatment because the information will be fresh in the PTA's mind.

4. Abbreviations should not be used because not everyone reading the note may know the meaning of the abbreviation. Many reading the note will not want to take the time to look up the meaning of abbreviations. Some may misinterpret the meaning (an abbreviation may have many meanings). Misinterpreting an abbreviation can cause harm to a patient and/or a delay in his or her treatment.

5. Many health care providers other than physical therapy–trained providers use some of the same treatment techniques that are used by PTs and PTAs. Putting the license or registration number after the signature identifies those treatments that were provided by physical therapy–trained personnel. This will help when medical records are researched to determine frequency of use and effectiveness of the treatment techniques.

CHAPTER 5   Review exercises are on page 73.

1. Subjective data consist of information that the patient, a family member, or representative of the patient tells the PT or PTA, and this information must be relevant to the problem and/or treatment.

2. Relevant subjective data consist of information that can influence the treatment or goal planning, prove treatment effectiveness or ineffectiveness, or describe a change in the patient's condition. Relevant information consists of the patient's medical history, environment and lifestyle, emotions and attitudes, goals or functional outcomes, unusual events or chief complaints, response to treatment, level of functioning, and pain.

3. Subjective data content can be grouped according to the categories of the relevant information listed in Question 2. Organizing the content into these categories makes reading and understanding the information easier than when the content is randomly organized and seems to ramble.

4. Use verbs that inform the reader that the information is being provided by the patient and that the patient is telling the therapist.

    You may wish to quote the patient to make the meaning clearer.

    Indicate which information comes from the patient and which information is provided by someone else.

    Any information about pain is subjective data.

5. Pain information is always included in the subjective data content because the patient is perceiving the pain, interpreting the sensation, and reporting or describing it to the therapist.

6. Students often write too much subjective information that is irrelevant to the problem or treatment. Students often make the mistake of failing to include pain information in the subjective data content.

CHAPTER 6   Review exercises are on page 87.

1. Objective data must consist of information that can be reproduced or observed by someone else with the same training.

2. Results of measurements and tests.
Description of the patient's function.
Description of the treatment provided.
Objective observations made by the PTA.

3. Results of tests and measurements must be documented consistent with the method of documentation in the PT's initial evaluation. It should be clear what is being tested or measured, the position of the patient, the starting and ending points, and the points of measurements, as appropriate.

4. In describing the patient's function, the PTA should paint a picture of the patient performing the activity. The description should include the activity, type of equipment or assistive devices used, speed, time or distance, number of repetitions, amount of weight, type of gait pattern, amount of assistance needed and why, the environment, and the quality of the patient's movement.

5. To be reproducible, the treatment description should give the type of treatment, specific machine or piece of equipment if appropriate, dosage, time, frequency, parameters or settings, position of patient, target tissue or treatment area, physiological response desired if appropriate, and purpose of the treatment.

6. Students commonly make two major mistakes when documenting objective data: (1) writing about what they did rather than discussing what the patient did and (2) rambling or failing to organize the information into topics.

CHAPTER 7   Review exercises are on page 103.

1. The PTA interprets the data to inform the reader as to the significance or importance of the data or why the data is documented. It answers the "so what?" question that the reader may be thinking when reading the data content. The PTA interprets the data to demonstrate to the reader the treatment effectiveness and the progress toward the treatment goals or functional outcomes. It is the rationale for the necessity of the physical therapy treatment.

2. The action of the function or goal.
Criteria that can be measured that determines when the goal is met.
A time period in which the goal or outcome should be accomplished.

3. The PTA cannot determine or write the long- or short-term functional outcomes of the physical therapy treatment. The PTA can confer with the PT and assist with the planning. The PTA can document progress toward and accomplishment of the outcomes and goals with evidence contained in the data in the progress note.

4. The interpretation of the data in the progress note is the most important content to most readers because it informs the reader whether the treatment is effective and whether the patient is making progress. This is what the insurance representative, physician, lawyer, and supervising PT want to know.

5. Change in the severity of the impairment.
Progress toward accomplishment of the goals or outcomes.
Lack of progress or treatment ineffectiveness with recommendations.
Inconsistencies in the subjective and objective data.

6. Impairment changes are documented by repeating tests and measurements or observations as they were performed and documented in the initial evaluation.

   Progress or lack of progress toward goals is documented (1) by renaming the outcomes or goals, or referring to their numbers as listed in the initial evaluation; and (2) by stating how much progress has been made (or not made) toward accomplishing those specific goals.

Subjective and objective data should refer to tests, measurements, and functional activities described in the initial evaluation. The inconsistencies should relate to this same information, not to information that is not discussed in the initial evaluation.

7. Making generalized statements such as "pt. tolerated treatment well" and not relating statement to specific information in the data.

Making statements about information that is not mentioned in the data portion of the note.

Talking about new information.

Forgetting to talk about the patient's progress toward improving the functional limitation that brought the patient to physical therapy. Forgetting to talk about the goals or outcomes listed in the initial evaluation.

CHAPTER 8   Review exercises are on page 115.

1. The plan section of the PT's initial evaluation lists the treatment planned to accomplish the goals or outcomes. It describes what will be done to decrease the severity of the impairment and to improve the patient's functional abilities. Each modality or activity listed has a treatment objective or statement as to its purpose. The plan indicates the frequency of treatment and a time period within which the treatment will be given (duration). The interim evaluation contains changes or modifications of the treatment plan, and the discharge evaluation discusses the treatment or follow-up activities needed in the future after discharge.

2. The PTA cannot design the treatment plan and cannot modify the plan. The PTA can assist the PT, provide relevant information, and make suggestions.

3. The content of the plan section of the progress note describes what will happen between the time the note was written and the next treatment session or what will happen at the next session. This section may report the number of remaining treatment sessions the patient is expected to complete. The plan content should include statements about working with the PT.

4. The plan statements provide evidence of PT–PTA teamwork by discussing intentions to consult with the PT, notify the PT, and/or make recommendations to the PT.

CHAPTER 9   Review exercises are on page 127.

1. Documenting telephone conversations such as referrals and requests for information about the patient's condition.

Documenting patient's refusal of treatment.

Completing an incident report.

2. Name of the person referring.

Name of the person calling in the referral if different from the person doing the referring.

Name of the PTA taking the call.

Name, address, and pertinent information about the client.

Details of the referral.

Date of the call.

Statement that the referral will be mailed to the caller for signature.

Statement that the PT will be notified.

3. If questions arise regarding any aspect of the referral, the persons involved in the telephone conversation can be contacted easily for clarification.

4. The rule of confidentiality is the ethical principle that all information about the patient, such as the treatment and the patient's condition, is confidential. Only the persons providing that

medical care are to have access to the information; anyone else must have permission from the patient to receive the information.

5. Give information about the client only to the persons for whom the client has signed a release of information form.
Keep the client's medical record in a location where unauthorized people cannot read it. Discuss the patient in private and only with persons authorized to have access to the information.

6. The release of information form is signed by the patient to authorize a person to receive medical information about the patient. This form protects the confidentiality of the patient by ensuring that the information goes only to those persons whom the patient agrees should know the information.

7. First determine why the patient is refusing treatment. Then explore with the patient alternatives or ideas that will include receiving the treatment and satisfying the patient. Explain the consequences of not receiving treatment. If the reason for refusal is valid or the patient persists in refusing, recognize the right of the patient to refuse, document this, and notify the PT.

8. A statement in the chart that the patient refused treatment; give the reason, report what the PTA did to encourage treatment, and state that the PT will be or was notified. This statement is placed in lieu of a progress note.

9. An incident is anything happening to the patient, an employee, or a visitor that is unusual, out of the ordinary, not part of routine or procedure, or inconsistent with treatment procedures; an accident or a situation that could cause an accident.

10. Name of the person involved in the incident, address, pertinent information.
Date of the incident.
Name and address of the eyewitness writing the incident report.
Names and addresses of other eyewitnesses.
Description and identification of equipment involved.
Objective, factual description of the incident.
Description of the action taken at the time of the incident.
Description of the status or condition of the person involved before and after the incident.
Description of the environmental conditions before and after the incident.

11. An incident report identifies situations that pose a danger to patients, employees, and visitors. Facilities have risk management procedures for correcting these situations to maintain a safe environment for everyone. The incident report policy requires a procedure for the provision of immediate medical care or action when an incident occurs. The report provides an objective record of the details if needed in the event of a litigation.

12. The incident report is kept in a separate file because it is confidential hospital information. The incident is documented in the patient's chart, but there should be no mention of the incident report in the medical record.

Answers to Practice Exercises

CHAPTER 2 Practice exercises begin on page 23.

1. The medical problem is **fractured right femur.**
   The PT musculoskeletal problem is **decreased strength in quadriceps.**
   The functional limitation is **unable to transfer independently in and out of bed or chair.**
   In the past, how would the treatment results have been documented?
   > By documenting the amount of strength of quadriceps gained.

   What is the recommended way to document treatment results?
   > By describing how the patient has improved in his or her ability to transfer in and out of bed and chair.

2. The medical diagnosis is **cerebral vascular accident.**
   The PT neuromusculoskeletal problem is **weakness and extensor hypertonus in the left lower extremity.**
   The functional limitation is **inability to climb stairs independently.**
   The treatment results should be documented by **describing the improvement in the patient's ability to climb stairs.**

3. The medical diagnosis is **incomplete spinal cord injury.**
   The neuromusculoskeletal PT problem is **lower-extremity paraparesis.**
   The functional limitation is **inability to stand.**
   The best way to document treatment results is by **describing the patient's improvement in his ability to stand.**

4. <u>PT</u>   Initial evaluation

   <u>PTA</u>   Progress notes

   <u>PTA</u>   Measurements results

   <u>PT</u>   Progress evaluation

   <u>PT</u>   Change in treatment plan

   <u>PTA</u>   Discharge summary with no interpretation or recommendations

   <u>PT</u>   Discharge evaluation

5. **Mr. Jones**
   Pathology is **fractured vertebra and severed spinal cord.**
   Impairment is **paralyzed legs.**
   Functional limitation is **inability to stand or walk.**
   Disability is **inability to play football and return to his profession.**

Sally

Pathology is **third-degree burns with scar tissue.**

Impairment is **scar tissue and limited ROM in fingers and wrists.**

Functional limitation is **inability to pick up and manipulate small objects.**

Disability is **inability to perform work that requires fine hand manipulation.**

Mrs. Williams

Pathology is **rheumatoid arthritis.**

Impairment is **limited ROM in knees and hips.**

Functional limitation is **inability to climb stairs or steps.**

Disability is **inability to live or function in an environment that contains stairs and steps.**

CHAPTER 3

Practice exercises begin on page 43.

1. *Example:*

   S: My car is saying "flap, flap, flap."

   O: I feel the car pulling to the right. After stopping at the side of the road, I get out and observe that the right front tire is flat. After preparing the car to change the flat, I cannot turn the bolts. I observe rust around them.

   A: Unable to meet goal to independently change flat tire. Need to seek help. Not able to go further in my car.

   P: Will walk to nearest house to call AAA for help.—Marianne Lukan

2. **Dx:** Multiple sclerosis.

   Pr: LE weakness limiting ability to sit ↔ stand and ambulate safely.

   Patient expresses frustration can't get up from couch without help, especially in evening.

   Gross MMT 3−/5 all LE muscle groups, 2/5 initial eval.

   Observed patient sitting in middle of couch.

   Patient sat at end of couch, scooted forward to edge, used couch arm to help push up.

   3rd trial able to sit to stand Ⓘ. Verbal cues to lean forward.

   Instructed patient to not sit on couch in evening when fatigued and weaker.

   Strength gain in LEs.

   Goal Ⓘ sit to stand met.

   Will visit patient 2 more times and schedule PT discharge evaluation.

3. **3-26-89**   **Dx:** Fx R femur, pinned 3-22-89.

   Pr: Limited RLE mobility and NWB.

   Pt. says he needs to be able to climb three flights of stairs to get to his apartment. Handrail on L going up. R ankle & foot edema. Circumference equals L foot & ankle measurements (see initial eval.). R knee flexion PROM 10–110° (15–100° last session). All R ankle AROM WNL. Pt. correctly demonstrated self knee ROM & gentle stretching exercises (see copy in chart). Pt. ambulated, NWB R, axillary crutches, Ⓘ, on grass and uneven sidewalk, 300 ft. RLE mobility progressing. Pt. has met his short-term goal of independent crutch walking on level and uneven ground. Will work on stair climbing next session. Will inform PT that pt. will be ready for discharge evaluation next session. _____

   —Confused Student, SPTA/Puzzled Therapist, PT (Lic. #420)

4.

Exercise	Set	Rep	Equipment	Assist
DX: R CVA with L hemiplegia				INITIAL DATE: 2-24-95
PRECAUTIONS: Broca's Aphasia, feeding tube				UPDATE: 3-25-95

DX: R CVA with L hemiplegia   INITIAL DATE: ____2-24-95____

PRECAUTIONS: Broca's Aphasia, feeding tube

UPDATE: ____3-25-95____

Exercise	Set	Rep	Equipment	Assist
Scapular protraction, supine L		5		Active assist
L elbow extension, supine		5		tap muscle
PROM/AAROM L UE & L LE	1	10		muscle belly
PRE R UED1 & D2 diagonals, supine	1	10	2# cuff wt	tapping
	1	10	3# cuff wt	verbal cues
	1	as many as he can, goal 4#		10 reps
Resistive active exercise R LE				
SLR, abduction sidelying, prone	2	10	5# cuff wt	verbal cues
knee flexion				
TKE long sitting	2	10	5# cuff wt	

Goals

1. Independent bed mobility
2. Independent unsupported sitting
3. Independent wheelchair mobility
4. Standing pivot transfer with
   minimum assist of 1

TDD:

TDP:

Patient's Name	Age	Sex	MD	PT	RM#	Units
Harry A	71	M	Smith	Jones	E123	12

Transfers bed <-> w/c, w/c <-> mat	Method	Assist	Other
table, w/c <-> toilet, w/c <->	stand pivot	maximum	Practice squat pivot transfer w/c <-> mat moving towards L
straight chair	to R side	x1	

Pregait/Gait

Amb x2 in //bars - max assist x2 - for wt shifting to L and knee control using temp AFO on L

Sitting balance in w/c with arms removed and in armless straight chair. Minimum assist x1. Work on head movement, eye
tracking, wt shifting, trunk rot.

W/c mobility - room to bathroom, room to dining room, to PT department, to OT, speech. Check seating/cushion,
L scapula protracted, arm on tray. Independent & brings self to department.

5.

TOTAL KNEE ARTHROPLASTY

	Date 8-8-95		Date 8-9-95		Date 8-10-95		Date 8-11-95		Date 8-12-95	
	am	pm	am	pm	am	pm	am	pm	am	pm
CPM Degrees	25	25	40	40	60	60	70	70	d/c by nursing	
CPM Time	1 hr on/1 hr off		same		same		same			
Knee ROM AA = Active Assist A = Active Supine			3 - 30	same	3 - 35	same	5 - 55	5 - 60	5 - 80	
Sitting			Pain, needs support		to 45	same	to 60	to 75	to 80	
Exercises: Isometrics Quads/Gluts/HS			Independent good coordination		Independent		same		I	
Ankle Pumps			Independent		Independent		same		I	
TKE					Independent		same		I	
SLR			Unable independent		Independent		min assist	Ind	I	
Active Knee Flex			Too painful to do		Independent		same		I	
Transfers: Bed Mobility			mod assist with leg		same		Independent		I	
Toilet/Commode									I	
Shower Seat									I	
Car Transfer									I	
Standing Pivot					yes		yes		yes	
Sliding Board										
Supine <--> Sit			mod assist knee supp		same		SBA		I	
Sit <--> Stand							Independent		I	
Balance: Sitting					good on edge of bed		same		I	
Standing			at side of bed		mod assist 1/walker				I	
Ambulation: Device			Too painful to start		walker		walker	crutches	crutches	
Weight Bearing			PWB R LE		PWB 50% body wt		PWB 75%		same	
Pattern									3 pt step thru	
Distance					few steps to chr/50'		50'x2	50'x1	125'	
Surface					level, tiled		tile,carpet	level	tile,carpet	
Assist					mod assist x1		SBA	min assist	Ind	
Stairs									SBA	
Blood Pressure					140/85 $\bar{a}$ 145/88 $\bar{p}$					
Pulse					72 bpm $\bar{a}$ 100 bpm $\bar{p}$					
Modalities	ice pack prn		continuous ice pack		same		d/c in am			
THERAPIST	Jennifer Nice, PT		Mary Jones, PTA		Mary Jones, PTA		Mary Jones, PTA		Mary Jones, PTA	

PHYSICAL THERAPY PROGRESS

PRECAUTIONS: Drain in place 8-8-95, 8-9-95 am, removed 8-9-95 pm

NAME: Earl

CHAPTER 4   Practice exercises begin on page 59.

1. **9/17/94**   **Dx:** Left total knee arthroplasty.

> **Pr:** Dependent in ambulation, right lower extremity weakness, partial weight bearing allowed.
>
> **S:** Patient's wife states he slept "poorly" last two nights. Minimal complaints of pain with exercise during treatment session.
>
> **O:** Patient transferred supine to sitting on right side of bed with moderate assist of one. Sat 5 minutes with complaints of dizziness. Gait training with front-wheeled walker, partial weight bearing on left, flat surface, 30 feet, moderate assist of one, 2 times with 5 minutes rest in between. Patient returned to bed for therapeutic exercise to left lower extremity: quadriceps sets, 10 repetitions, 5-second hold with strong contraction; straight leg raises, 10 repetitions with external rotation to decrease 10° lag. Active range of motion left knee 10–50°, passive range of motion 0–60°.
>
> **A:** Increased range of motion, increased distance. Patient making gains even though not able to sleep well. Patient expected to achieve short-term goal of increased range of motion, increased strength, and minimal assist gait.
>
> **P:** Continue with gait training and therapeutic exercise. Begin stair ambulation in afternoon 9/18/94.—John Thomas, PTA

2. 1. No date and signature.
    2. Many open spaces where someone could insert information or falsify the record.
    3. Incorrect grammar and spelling.

3. 1. Not full legal signature and no title.
    2. Note not brief, some information not relevant to the problem of treatment.
    3. Not clear (e.g., what does "lots of cheating" mean?).
    4. Spelling and punctuation incorrect.
    5. Error not initialed and dated.

4. **9-4-90:**   **Dx:** Psoriasis both arms.

> **Pr:** Difficulty sleeping and concentrating due to severe itching.
>
> **S:** Pt. states R elbow itches a lot. States his knees feel stiff, has trouble getting up out of his favorite chair. _____
>
> **O:** Saw pt. 4 times. Did ultraviolet treatments to both arms to dry up the sores. No more rash on the L forearm._____
>
> **A:** Pt. tolerating treatment well._____
>
> **P:** Continue per PT's initial plan.
>
> —Marianne Lukan, PT

5. **11-17-92**   **Dx:** L CVA.

> **Pr:** Weakness in RUE & RLE with unsafe ambulation and dependent in ADLs.
>
> Pt. states not doing exercises at home, has not been going out to church or club meetings because she is afraid of falling. Pt. states she has always been active and wishes she could go to her bridge club meetings. L hand extremely purple! Can't bear wt. on hand due to stiffness in fingers, decreased ROM in all finger joints. Can't push on hand to get up off of floor. Isometrics to shoulder, with substitution by leaning trunk. ~~PROM~~ ^{11-17-92 ml} AAROM to all motions of the shoulder, elbow, forearm, and wrist, 10 reps each in supine position. Independent supine to sit if pt. rolls to R elbow for support and pushes with L hand to get up. Pt. has difficulty comprehending, is impatient, is uncooperative. Will continue treatment 3×/week per PT's plan.
>
> —Marianne Lukan, PT

CHAPTER 5   Practice exercises begin on page 75.

1. <u>SD</u> Pt. states she has a clear understanding of her disease and her prognosis.

   <u>SD</u> Pt. expresses surprise that the ice massage relaxed her muscle spasm.

   <u>Pr</u> Muscle spasms L lumbar paraspinals with sitting tolerance limited to 10 min.

   <u>SD</u> Pt. describes tingling pain down back of R leg to heel.

   <u>Pr</u> Dependent in ADLs due to flaccid paralysis in R upper and lower extremities.

   <u>SD</u> Sue states her L ear hurts.

   <u>Pr</u> Unable to reach behind back due to limited ROM in R shoulder int. rot.

   <u>SD</u> Reports he must be able to return to work as a welder.

   <u>Pr</u> Laceration of R vastus medialis.

   <u>Pr</u> Paraplegic 2° SCI T_{12} and dependent in wheelchair transfers.

   <u>SD</u> States Hx of RA since 1980.

   <u>SD</u> Pt. denies pain c̄ cough.

   <u>SD</u> States injury occurred December 31, 1994.

   <u>SD</u> SPTA c/o he has to sit for 2 hours in the PTA lectures.

   <u>Pr</u> Grip strength weakness and inability to turn doorknobs to open doors due to carpal tunnel syndrome.

   <u>SD</u> Describes his pain as "burning."

   <u>Pr</u> Unable to sit due to decubitus over sacrum.

   <u>Pr</u> Unable to feed self due to limited elbow flexion.

   <u>SD</u> Pt. rates her pain a 4 on an ascending scale of 1–10.

   <u>SD</u> States able to sit through a 2-hour movie last night.

2. <u>Pr</u> <u>Muscle spasms</u> L lumbar paraspinals with sitting tolerance limited to 10 min.

   <u>Pr</u> Dependent in ADLs due to <u>flaccid paralysis</u> in R upper and lower extremities.

   <u>Pr</u> Unable to reach behind back due to <u>limited ROM</u> in R shoulder int. rot.

   <u>Pr</u> <u>Laceration</u> of R vastus medialis.

   <u>Pr</u> <u>Paraplegic</u> 2° SCI T_{12} and dependent in wheelchair transfers.

   <u>Pr</u> <u>Grip strength weakness</u> and inability to turn doorknobs to open doors due to carpal tunnel syndrome.

   <u>Pr</u> Unable to sit due to <u>decubitus</u> over sacrum.

   <u>Pr</u> Unable to feed self due to <u>limited elbow flexion</u>.

   <u>SD</u> Pt. <u>states</u> she has a clear understanding of her disease and her prognosis.

   <u>SD</u> Pt. <u>expresses</u> surprise that the ice massage relaxed her muscle spasm.

   <u>SD</u> Pt. <u>describes</u> tingling pain down back of R leg to heel.

   <u>SD</u> Sue <u>states</u> her L ear hurts.

   <u>SD</u> <u>Reports</u> he must be able to return to work as a welder.

   <u>SD</u> <u>States</u> Hx of RA since 1980.

   <u>SD</u> Pt. <u>denies</u> pain c̄ cough.

   <u>SD</u> <u>States</u> injury occurred December 31, 1994.

   <u>SD</u> SPTA <u>c/o</u> he has to sit for 2 hours in the PTA lectures.

   <u>SD</u> Describes his pain as "burning."

   <u>SD</u> Pt. <u>rates</u> her pain a 4 on an ascending scale of 1–10.

   <u>SD</u> <u>States</u> able to sit through a 2-hour movie last night.

Medical diagnoses:
Laceration
SCI
RA
Carpal tunnel syndrome
Decubitus

3. **Mistakes:**

1. Used a pain scale, whereas the PT used a body drawing in the initial evaluation. One cannot compare a pain scale with a body drawing to document treatment effectiveness.

2. Talked about pain in the objective data section or did not write that the patient states or reports pain when lying propped on elbows or reports no pain in buttock area.

6-3-94:   **Dx:** Disc protrusion L4,5.

Pr: Muscle spasms lumbar paraspinals with limited sitting and sleeping tolerance, difficulty with ADLs, and unable to perform work tasks.

Patient states she was able to sit through 30 minutes of "The Young and The Restless" soap opera yesterday. Marked body drawing with pain located in right low back, but not in buttock area. Colored markings green instead of red as in initial evaluation, indicating decreased pain intensity. See body drawing in chart. Before traction reported inability to tolerate lying propped on elbow because of pain in low back. Patient has received 4 treatment sessions. Decrease in muscle tone palpable after 10 minute massage to right lumbar paraspinal muscles, prone position over one thin pillow. Able to lie propped on elbows 5 minutes following 10 minutes, prone, static pelvic traction, 70 lb. Correctly performed lumbar extension exercises 1, 2, and 3 of home exercise program (see copy in chart) and observed consistently using correct sitting posture with lumbar roll. Patient required frequent verbal cuing for correct body mechanics while performing 10 reps (3 reps in initial eval.) of circuit of job simulation activities consisting of bed making, rolling and moving 30-lb (10-lb in initial eval.) dummy "patient" in bed, pivot transferring the dummy, and wheelchair handling. She did 10 back arches between each task without reminders. Patient has reached 30-minute sitting tolerance goal, is independent with home exercise program and compliant with techniques for controlling the protrusion. Progress toward outcome of return to work is 60% with more consistent use of correct body mechanics and ability to lift 50-lb dummy required. Patient to continue treatment sessions 33/week for 2 more weeks per PT's initial plan. Will notify PT that interim evaluation is scheduled for 6-7-94.

—Sue Smith, PTA, Lic. #0003

4. <u>Yes</u>   Client stated her dog was hit by a car last night and she felt too depressed today to do her exercises.

<u>Yes</u>   Client reported he progressed his exercises to 50 push-ups yesterday.

<u>No</u>   Patient's daughter stated she traveled from Iowa, where it has been raining for 2 weeks.

<u>No</u>   Patient states he does not like the hospital food and is hungry for some Dairy Queen.

<u>Yes</u>   Patient rates her pain a 4 on an ascending scale of 1–7.

<u>Yes</u>   Patient states she is now able to reach the second shelf of her kitchen cupboard to reach for a glass.

<u>Yes</u>   Patient reports he had this same tingling discomfort in his right foot 3 years ago.

<u>Yes</u>	Client reports experiencing an aching in his "elbow bone" after the ultrasound treatment yesterday.
<u>No</u>	Patient says she has 10 grandchildren and 4 great grandchildren.
<u>Yes</u>	Client states she forgot to tell the PT that she loves to bowl.
<u>No</u>	Client reports that "Northern Exposure" is his favorite TV program.
<u>Yes</u>	Client reports he sat in his fishing boat 3 hours and caught a 7-lb Northern this week end.
<u>Yes</u>	Client states he played golf yesterday for the first time since his back injury.
<u>No</u>	Client states he shot a 56 in golf.
<u>Yes</u>	Client states she cannot turn her head to look over her shoulder to back the car out of the garage.
<u>No</u>	Patient's mother wants to know when her son will come out of the coma.
<u>No</u>	Client reports he wishes he had not been drinking beer the night of his accident.
<u>Yes</u>	Patient describes his flight of stairs with 10 steps, a landing, then 5 more steps and the railing on the right when going up.
<u>No</u>	Client wishes it would rain as her prize roses are dying.
<u>Yes</u>	Patient states, "I'm going to Macy's to shop and have lunch today." (Patient is 89 years old and is a resident in a long-term care facility in a small town in Ohio. She has been placed on some new medication.)

CHAPTER 6 Practice exercises begin on page 89.

1. <u>SD</u> Pt. c/o pain with prolonged sitting.

<u>OD</u> Decubitus on sacrum measures 3 cm from L outer edge to R outer edge.

<u>OD</u> Pt. ambulates with ataxic gait, 10 ft, max assist of 2 to prevent fall.

<u>OD</u> R knee flexion PROM 30–90°.

<u>OD</u> Ambulates c̄ standard walker, PWB L, bed to bathroom (20 ft), tiled surface, min assist 1× verbal cuing for gait pattern.

<u>SD</u> Pt. states he is fearful of crutch walking.

<u>Pr</u> Limited ROM in L shoulder 2° to Fx greater tubercle of humerus and unable to put on winter coat without help.

<u>SD</u> c/o itching in scar R knee.

<u>OD</u> Transfers: supine ↔ sit c̄ min. assist 1× for strength.

<u>Pr</u> Unable to feed self with L hand due to limited elbow ROM 2° Fx L olecranon process.

<u>OD</u> AROM WNL bil. LEs.

<u>OD</u> Pt. demonstrated adequate knee flexion during initial swing c̄ verbal cuing p̄ hamstring exercises.

<u>Pr</u> Dependent in bed mobility due to dislocated R hip.

<u>SD</u> Expresses concern over lack of progress.

<u>OD</u> L shoulder flexion PROM 0–100°, lat. rot. PROM 0–40°.

<u>SD</u> Kathy reports PTA courses are easy.

<u>OD</u> Pt. pivot transfers, NWB R, bed ↔ w/c, max assist of 2 for strength, balance, NWB cuing.

<u>SD</u> Pt. rates L knee pain 5/10 when going up stairs.

<u>OD</u> LUE circumference at 3 cm superior to olecranon process is 12 cm.

<u>OD</u> BP 125/80 mmHg, pulse 78 BPM, regular, strong.

2. <u>Pr</u> <u>Limited ROM</u> in L shoulder 2° to Fx greater tubercle of humerus and ⟨unable to put on winter coat without help⟩

   <u>Pr</u> ⟨Unable to feed self with L hand⟩ due to <u>limited elbow ROM</u> 2° Fx L olecranon process.

   <u>Pr</u> ⟨Dependent in bed mobility⟩ due to <u>dislocated R hip.</u>

<u>SD</u> Pt. <u>c/o</u> pain with prolonged sitting.

<u>SD</u> Pt. <u>states</u> he is fearful of crutch walking.

<u>SD</u> <u>c/o</u> itching in scar R knee.

<u>SD</u> <u>Expresses</u> concern over lack of progress.

<u>SD</u> Kathy <u>reports</u> PTA courses are easy.

<u>SD</u> Pt. <u>rates</u> L knee pain 5/10 when going up stairs.

<u>OD</u> Decubitus on sacrum <u>measures 3 cm</u> from L outer edge to R outer edge.

<u>OD</u> Pt. <u>ambulates with ataxic gait, 10 ft max assist of 2</u> to prevent fall.

<u>OD</u> R knee flexion <u>PROM 30–90°</u>

<u>OD</u> Ambulates c̄ <u>standard walker, PWB L, bed to bathroom (20 ft), tiled surface, min. assist 1× for balance, verbal cuing for gait pattern.</u>

<u>OD</u> Transfers: <u>supine ↔ sit c̄ min. assist for strength.</u>

<u>OD</u> AROM <u>WNL</u> bil. LEs.

<u>OD</u> Pt. <u>demonstrated adequate knee flexion during initial swing</u> c̄ verbal cuing p̄ hamstring exercises.

<u>OD</u> L shoulder flexion <u>PROM 0–100°, lat. rot. PROM 0–40°.</u>

<u>OD</u> Pt. <u>pivot transfers, NWB R, bed ↔ w/c, max assist of 2 for strength, balance, NWB cuing.</u>

<u>OD</u> LUE <u>circumference at 3 cm superior to olecranon process is 12 cm.</u>

<u>OD</u> <u>BP 125/80 mmHg, pulse 78 BPM, regular, strong.</u>

Medical diagnoses:

   Decubitus

   Fx greater tubercle of humerus

   Fx left olecranon process

   Dislocated hip

3. 1. Nothing wrong, documentation complete.
    2. Measurement scale not consistent with initial eval. Used inches in progress note vs. centimeters in initial evaluation.
    3. Right or left hip? Passive or active ROM? Which motion? The hip has six motions. No starting point for the measurement. What position was patient in?
    4. Right or left? Measurement scale not the same as used in PT's initial evaluation.
    5. No starting point for the measurement. It should read 0–20°.
    6. Measurement sites not specific enough, no position of patient.
    7. Blood pressure should be in mmHg, pulse in BPM, no position of patient, do not know when the measurements were taken (exercise or resting).
    8. All measurements recorded in inches except for one, recorded in centimeters.
    9. Nothing wrong, documentation complete.
    10. The starting point of the measurements not documented. Active or passive motion?
    11. Nothing wrong. Documentation complete.
    12. Measurement landmarks not documented.
    13. An estimate or judgment by observation. Not everyone will make the same judgment. Measurement technique not described.
    14. No measurement technique described.
    15. Nothing wrong. Documentation complete.

4. 1. Cannot reproduce. Need type of US, more specific target tissue, position of patient, time, purpose.
    2. Cannot reproduce. Need type of massage, patient position, purpose, more specific treatment area, time.
    3. Can reproduce. Documentation complete.
    4. Cannot reproduce. Need list or type of exercises, more specific as to treatment area (e.g., which motion?), patient position, repetitions.
    5. Cannot reproduce. Need type of traction equipment (static or intermittent), pounds, on/off time, duration, patient position, which muscles.
    6. Cannot reproduce. Need to know purpose.
    7. Can reproduce. Documentation complete. Assume all information is in written instructions in copy in chart.
    8. Cannot reproduce. Need dosage and time.
    9. Cannot reproduce. Need patient position, parameters or settings, electrode size, number, and placement, time or duration.
    10. Can reproduce. Documentation complete.

5. 1. Following instructions, patient safely and independently ambulated no wt. bearing on right with axillary crutches 100 ft on tiled and carpeted level surfaces, was able to sit down and rise from bed, chair, toilet, and transfer in and out of car. She managed a flight of stairs with crutches and railing (on right going up) with verbal cuing. She safely managed two steps and curbs with crutches. Patient was provided with written crutch-walking instructions for reminders. See copy in chart.
    2. Client performed circuit of brick layer job simulation activities to practice correct body mechanics 20 minutes, 15 repetitions for goal of returning to work. Client observed consistently using correct body mechanics and maintaining lumbar curve when lifting bricks and spreading mortar, but required verbal cuing to correct his tendency to bend and twist at the waist when wheeling and turning the wheelbarrow.
    3. Patient practiced sliding board transfers from wheelchair ↔ toilet 3×, requiring frequent verbal cuing for safety precautions, and progressing from maximum assist to help push across the board to minimum assist on third transfer from chair to toilet. Moderate assist needed on third attempt to push from toilet back into chair.
    4. Patient ambulated with wide-based quad cane on left from bed to bathroom, to window, to hall in front of room, to wheelchair next to bed 5× with 2 minutes rest in chair between each circuit. He required minimum assist for wt. shifting to the right first 3 times, but demonstrated independent wt. shifting during the 4th and 5th walks. Patient independently recovered slight loss of balance 3×.

CHAPTER 7   Practice exercises begin on page 105.

1. **Situation A:**

    LTGs: At anticipated discharge date in 1 month:

    2. Patient will be able to manage two steps with an assistive device and a railing and to manage car transfers for next visit to the doctor in 4 weeks.

    STGs: 1. Pt. will consistently move up and down in bed and roll from side to side with SBA in 2 weeks.

    2. Pt. will consistently roll to L side and reach for telephone and call bell with SBA in 3 weeks.

    3. Pt. will consistently move from supine to sitting on edge of bed and return to supine position with minimal assist of 1 to help swing L leg into bed in 1 week.

    4. Pt. will consistently move from sitting to standing and back to sitting from bed, toilet, wheelchair, standard chair with minimum assist of 1 for balance control and even weight bearing cuing in 2 weeks.

5. Using a quad cane, pt. will <u>consistently</u> ⟨ambulate⟩ <u>bed to bathroom, and to meals with moderate assist of 1 for balance control and gait posture cuing</u> ~~in one week~~.

Situation B:

LTGs: At anticipated discharge ~~in 20 days~~, patient will ⟨transfer and ambulate⟩ <u>independently</u> for return to home.

1. Patient will <u>independently and consistently</u> ⟨move⟩ <u>from sit to stand and stand to sit using elevated toilet seat, and all other surfaces no lower than 18 inches.</u>

2. Patient will <u>independently and consistently</u> ⟨walk⟩ <u>with a single-end cane on all surfaces and in the community.</u>

STGs: 1. Pt. will <u>consistently</u> be able ⟨to sit to stand and return⟩ <u>with standby assist (SBA) of 1 if boost is needed from edge of bed, elevated toilet seat, wheelchair, and standard dining room chair</u> ~~in 10 days~~.

2. Pt. will <u>consistently</u> be able to ⟨ambulate⟩ <u>using a single-end cane for balance on tiled and carpeted level surfaces, to bathroom and dining room for meals with SBA of 1 for balance control</u> ~~in 10 days~~.

2. 1. Increase right knee PROM to 0–90° in 1 week.

In 1 week, pt. will be able to use 0–90° PROM in right knee to sit in narrow theater seat aisle for 30 minutes in preparation for return to work as a movie critic.

2. Sit unsupported and independently on edge of bed for 5 minutes in 3 days.

In 3 days, pt. will be able to sit independently and without support on the edge of the bed for 5 minutes to eat her afternoon snack.

3. Ambulate 30 ft on tiled level surface, using standard walker, partial weight bearing on left, with standby assist for verbal cuing for gait pattern in 4 days.

In 4 days, pt. will ambulate with standard walker for partial weight bearing on left, from bed to bathroom, with nursing assistant for standby assist for verbal cuing for safety.

4. Increase strength of left hip abductors from 3/5 to 4/5 in 3 weeks.

In 3 weeks, patient's left hip abductors will have increased strength (4/5) to allow pt. to ambulate two city blocks without an assistive device and without a left trunk lean.

5. Decrease pain rating on pain scale from 6/10 to 3/10 in 4 treatment sessions.

After 4 treatment sessions, pt. will rate pain 3/10 while demonstrating smooth movements and even weight bearing when performing nursing assistant job simulation tasks with proper body mechanics.

6. Will be able to safely perform job tasks so as to be able to return to work in 1 month.

Patient will be able to lift and carry 50-lb boxes from conveyor belt to pallet and stack boxes on the pallet, using safe body mechanics and back protection techniques as required for his return to work in 1 month.

3. **4-17-94**   **Dx:** R Colles' fracture, healed, cast removed.

Pr: Restricted ROM in wrist with inability to open doors, limited ability to grasp and pull for dressing activities.

S: <u>Pt. reports able to put on panty hose today without help from husband and turned bathroom doorknob to open the door.</u>

O: Pt. has been seen 2×. Pt. performed AROM exercises R forearm pronation/supination while in arm whirlpool, 110°, 20 min to increase circulation and increase extensibility to R wrist tissues to prepare for stretching exercises. Contract–relax stretching techniques, 5 reps each, to increase pronation, supination and wrist extension ROM, sitting with forearm supported on table. Pt. correctly demonstrated home exercise program for strengthening finger flexion, wrist flexion and extension, forearm pronation and supination (see copy in chart). <u>ROM today vs. 4-10-94:</u>

	4-17-95	4-10-95
R pronation	0–50°	0–40°
R supination	0–70°	0–60°
Wrist extension	0–30°	0–20°

<u>Grip strength 20 lb today, 10 lb 4-10-95. Pt. turned door handles and opened all inside doors in the clinic using R hand, but unable to turn handle and open door to outside. Able to grasp rope on scale and pull, exerting 3-lb force (2-lb 4-10-95).</u>

A: Strengthening and stretching treatment procedures effective in increasing strength and ROM, improving progress toward goals of independent dressing activities and ability to open all types of doors.

P: To see pt. on 4-24-95 and notify PT discharge eval. to be 4-31-95. Will work on opening outside doors next visit.

—Sally Citizen, PTA, Lic. #5631

4. 1. No evidence to support statement that quads have decreased strength. Need some measurement of quadriceps strength or comparison of ability to do the exercises with performance in previous sessions or initial evaluation.

No evidence to support statement about decreased control of knee extension with exercise. Need description of quality of the movement during exercise in objective section.

No comments about how the knee control and the quadriceps strength relate to the patient's ambulation. No comment about ambulation goals, treatment goals, or progress toward any outcomes that may be mentioned in the initial evaluation.

No comments as to whether or not E-stim treatment was effective for muscle reeducation.

5. **1-20-87**   **Dx:** Orthostatic hypotension 2° SCI C7

Pr: Unable to tolerate upright sitting.

S: Pt. continues to c/o dizziness when he attempts sitting.

O: Pt. has had 3 sessions on the tilt table to develop tolerance for upright sitting. First session BP dropped from 130/80 mmHg to 90/50 mmHg p̄ 10 min. at 40° elevation. Today BP dropped from 130/80 mmHg ā tx to 100/60 mm Hg p̄ 15 min. on tilt table at 50°. BP 125/75 mmHg 5 min p̄ pt. returned to supine position.

A: Progress toward goal of upright sitting for 30 min is 50%. Severity of orthostatic hypotension decreasing. Blood pressure more stable with less drop than previous treatment sessions and with appropriate recovery.

6. **11-2-85**   **Pr:** Open wound due to 2nd-degree burn on L gluteus medius, not able to sit with even wt. bearing.

Pt: Reports itching around edge of wound. Pt. sat in whirlpool 100°, 20 min for wound debridement and to increase circulation for healing, sterile technique dressing change. No eschar, edges pink, 1 tsp. drainage, clear, odorless. Diameter R outer edge to L outer edge: 4 cm today compared to $4\frac{3}{4}$ cm 10-31-85. Treatment is effective for goal to enhance wound healing process and closing for proper sitting. No evidence of infection.

CHAPTER 8   Practice exercises begin on page 117.

1. **1-20-87**   **Dx:** Orthostatic hypotension 2° SCI C$_7$.

Pr: Unable to tolerate upright sitting.

S: Pt. continues to c/o dizziness when he attempts sitting.

O: Pt. has had 3 sessions on the tilt table to develop tolerance for upright sitting. First session BP dropped from 130/80 mmHg to 90/50 mmHg p̄ 10 min at 40°elevation. Today BP dropped from 130/80 mmHg ā tx to 100/60 mmHg p̄ 15 min on tilt table at 50°. BP 125/75 mmHg 5 min p̄ pt returned to supine position.

A: Progress toward goal of upright sitting for 30 min is 50%. Severity of orthostatic hypotension decreasing. Blood pressure more stable with less drop than previous treatment sessions and with appropriate recovery.

P: Will continue tilt-table treatment bid per PT's plan until pt. tolerates 70° for 20 min then consult PT about when to try sitting in chair with back that reclines.

—Kathy A. Student, SPTA/Marianne Lukan, PT Lic. #xxx

2. **11-2-85   Pr:** Open wound due to 2nd-degree burn on L gluteus medius, not able to sit with even wt. bearing.

Pt. reports itching around edge of wound. Pt. sat in whirlpool 100°, 20 min for wound debridement and to increase circulation for healing, sterile technique dressing change. No eschar, edges pink, 1 tsp. drainage, clear, odorless. Diameter R outer edge to L outer edge: 4 cm today compared to 4¾ cm 10-31-85. Treatment is effective for goal to enhance wound healing process and closing for proper sitting. No evidence of infection. Will continue treatment daily per PT's plan until open area measures 2 cm and consult PT about time to begin ambulation.

Jerry A. Student, SPTA/Marianne Lukan, PT Lic. #xxx

3. 2. Exercises, including home program, for hip abductor muscles to <u>strengthen to grade 5/5.</u>

3. Home program of structured, progressive walking and stair climbing activities to <u>increase tolerance to the activities without aggravating the bursitis.</u> 3×/week and 2×/week = frequencies; 2 weeks = short-term duration; 1 month = long-term duration.

1. Exercises to strengthen all extremities <u>to aid transfers and ambulation.</u> Exercise plan to include home program.

2. Training and practice for transfers from <u>all types of surfaces as required in the home.</u>

3. Gait training with platform walker on level tiled and carpeted surfaces and one step <u>as required in the home.</u>

4. Home assessment visit to clarify needs <u>for transfer and gait training planning.</u>

5. Educate patient and family on hip protection and safety precautions for <u>safe functioning in the home.</u> bid = frequency; 2 weeks = duration.

1. Home program of exercises to <u>increase ROM and strength of L elbow and hip</u> in preparation for ambulation with cane and independent ADLs.

2. Transfer and ambulation training with progression of assistive devices appropriate for <u>safe change from platform walker to goal of single-end cane.</u>

3. Ambulation training <u>on grass and dock using assistive device.</u>

4. Stair climbing training with assistive device and railing in <u>home and into motor home.</u>
3×/week and 2×/week = frequencies; 2 weeks and 1 week = short-term durations; 3 weeks = long-term duration.

CHAPTER 9   Practice exercises begin on page 129.

1. **Name:** Janet Smith   **Room #:** 102 **MR #:** 2001 **Date:** 11/15/95

Pt. has orders for PT daily for strengthening exercises, transfer training, and gait training with walker. She declined treatment today, stating her RLE was "too sore and swollen from being up in wheelchair too long." Writer notes T.E.D.s socks on RLE with minimal edema at lateral malleolus, LEs elevated in bed at this time. Nurse's note reflects pt.'s request for increased Tylenol, which is medication provided pt. as needed. Encouraged pt. to perform isometric LE exercises previously instructed on while in bed. Plan to see for treatment tomorrow.

—Diane Palmstein, PTA/Mary Smith, PT

2.

PREDISPOSING CONDITIONS
Diagnosis: Fx ® hip, repaired with prothesis
Mental Status (i.e., Oriented, Alert/Confused, etc.): – Alert oriented –
List pertinent medications if applicable: Tylenol prn
Follow-Up Measures to Incident: monitor ® buttock pain complaints. Resume PT 12-2-95

Was a Medical Device Involved? ☐ Yes ☒ No   **Manufacturer's Name and Address (If Available on Equipment or Packaging):**

Type_____   Model No. _____

Serial No. _____   Lot No. _____

Incident Reported By: Marianne Lukas   **Title:** PTA

Date of Report: 12-1-95	**Signature & Title of Person Preparing Report:** Marianne Lukas PTA

Reviewed by DON:_____ (Signature)   **Reviewed by Administrator:**_____ (Signature)

Date:_____ **Charted:** ☐ Yes ☐ No   **Date:**_____

Reviewed by Medical Director:_____ **Date:**_____ (Signature or Initials)

DO NOT WRITE BELOW THIS LINE—TO BE COMPLETED BY ADMINISTRATOR/DON

Vulnerable Adult Report Made? Yes ☐   No ☐

Incident Reported To (Circle as many of the following as applicable.):

Local Welfare Agency   **Local Police Department**   **County Sheriff's Office**   **Office of Health Facility Complaints**

Other (Explain)_____

Date Report Called In (Within 5 Days):_____   **Approximate Time:**_____ ☐ a.m. ☐ p.m.

Name of Person Spoken to:_____   **Reported By:**_____

Date Report Mailed:_____   **To Whom:**_____

incident.rep

ABC HEALTH CENTER
INCIDENT REPORT

Resident/Visitor #1: Mr. X	Resident/Visitor #2: NA
Address: Room 201	Address:
Phone #: DOB 07/08/20	Phone #: DOB
Date: 12/01/95 Time 10:20 (am)/pm	Location of Incident: Room 201

Description of Incident: Pt is transfering from wheelchair to bed with a walker and with PTA on ® side holding transfer belt. During pivot, pt's ® knee buckles. PTA guides pt down onto the bed but the bed rolls back. PTA lowers pt to floor and rests pt's head and back against the PTA. Pt is in a semi reclined position with both legs straight out in front. PTA calls for help.

Assessment: Describe injury (if any) in detail: Pt ⊖ pain in ® buttocks, denies pain in ® hip or leg. No injury identified by physician.

Name/Title of All Witnesses:	Safety Measures in Use:
Marianne Lukas PTA	Transfer Belt: X
	Siderails:
	Restraint: _____ Type: _____

Intervention: None Required _____   At Facility X

Describe: Jane Doe RN and Tom Jones NA assisted PTA in lifting Mr. X from floor to bed. Dr. Young examined pt. No injury identified, but pt may have bumped buttocks on bed siderail. Pt to remain in bed and RN will monitor skin condition and pain complaints for remainder of the day.

Resident #1 Mr. X

Hospitalized: Yes___ No X	Date NA Time____am/pm	Hospital NA
Physician Name: Dr Young	Notified by: Jane Doe RN Date 12-1-95 Time 10:30 (am)/pm	
Family Name: Mrs. X	Notified by: Jane Doe RN Date 12-1-95 Time 11:00 (am)/pm	

Resident #2   NA

Hospitalized: Yes___ No___	Date_____ Time____am/pm	Hospital_____
Physician Name:	Notified by: Date_____ Time____am/pm	
Family Name:	Notified by: Date_____ Time____am/pm	

Safety lesson: Always lock brakes on wheeled beds.

CHAPTER 10   Practice exercises begin on page 145.

   1. **Pr:** Pt. has a decubitus over L lat. malleolus interfering with ability to wear proper shoe for ambulation.

     S: She states, "It is Christmas and I don't have my shopping done."

     O: Observed pt. scratching at her wound dressings. Wound dressing half off upon arrival to dept. Wound measures 3 cm horizontally across outer edge to outer edge (4 cm initial eval.), loose necrotic tissue, no drainage. Foot whirlpool 104°F, loose tissue dislodged, and dressings changed.

     A: 50% progress toward goal of clean, healing wound to prepare for ambulation.

     P: Will consult PT re: designing wrap over bandage to keep pt. from pulling dressing loose.

     Pr: Pt is 82 YO c̄ terminal CA.

     Subjective data: Pt. states he wants to go home. Pt.'s wife says she cannot care for pt. at home.

     Objective data: Gluteus maximus and quads 3/5. Major mm groups in LEs 3/5 to 4/5 strength range. Pt. demonstrated 3 reps each of LE strengthening exercises to be performed in the ward with wife's help (see copy in chart). Maximum assist for transfer bed ↔ commode ↔ w/c. He needs max. assistance for sit ↔ stand for strength to get up and for control when sitting down. Pt. ambulated 3× the length of the // bars (about 30 ft) c̄ min. assist for sense of security with verbal cues for posture and heel–toe stepping.

     Interpretation of the data: Pt. is not independent in ADLs due to muscle weaknesses.

     Plan: Will continue to work to ↑ mm strength and try sliding board transfers this PM.

   2. <u>SD:</u> Pt. reports pain relief several hours after treatment.

     <u>OD</u> Performed Codman's exercises with 2-lb wt. to distract shoulder.

     <u>OD</u> Electrode placed 2 inches above R elbow crease line.

     <u>Pr</u> R hemiplegia with spasticity and dependence for transfers and ambulation.

     <u>P</u> Will instruct in proper stair climbing next session.

     <u>OD</u> Missed 2 of his last 5 treatment sessions due to illness one day and refusal the other.

     <u>SD</u> C/o pain in RLE.

     <u>OD</u> Recommended family install railing on wall along stairs for safety.

     <u>ID</u> Goal met for child to roll side-lying to supine and prone 1/3 trials at least 3× in 2 months to improve mobility.

     <u>SD</u> Had terrible headache last night.

     <u>P</u> Will await further orders from physician.

     <u>OD</u> Pt. able to demonstrate home exercise program with good form.

     <u>SD</u> Pain intensity increased from 5 to 6/7.

     <u>OD</u> Requires moderate assist to get up from wheelchair and to lift legs back into bed.

     <u>SD</u> States he needs to lift a maximum of 70 lb from floor to conveyor belt.

     <u>OD</u> Performed 10 reps of UED1 exercises on the R using red Thera-Band and 20 reps of same exercise on the L with blue Thera-Band.

     <u>OD</u> Ambulated with forceful knee hyperextension during stance phase.

     <u>SD</u> My goal is to play golf.

     <u>Pr</u> Atrophy of quads and gastrocs limiting ability to manage stair climbing.

     <u>P</u> Will take standard walker to patient's home next visit.

__OD__ Wrist flexors 3/5, extensors 2/5 strength.

__SD__ Mother stated child rolled supine to prone last night.

__OD__ Decreased muscle tone palpable following massage.

__ID__ Progress toward goal of independent car transfers and community ambulation 80%.

__OD__ Pt. squats with narrow base of support and rounded low back, placing object in front of knees.

3. **3-26-89** **Pr:** R foot edema.

Says he needs to be able to climb three flights of stairs to get to his apartment. Handrail on L going up. Circumference equal L foot measurements. R knee flexion 10–110°. Pt. crutch walked NWB, 300 ft on grass outside c̄ no assistance. Pt. showing good progress in LE mobility. Pt. has met his short-term goal of independent crutch walking. Will work on stair climbing next session.

—Jim Jones, PTA

Pr does not have functional limitation. Pr does not relate to the treatment.

Legal guidelines followed.

Subjective data: correct.

Objective data: Cannot duplicate measurements of circumference because the measurement landmarks and position of patient are not documented. Position of patient for ROM measurements not described. We don't know whether measurements are consistent with initial evaluation, and ROM measurements are not compared with previous measurements. Ambulation description doesn't tell reader the type of crutches or how the pt.'s posture looked.

Interpretation of the data: No evidence to support the conclusion that LE mobility has improved. Note doesn't record any treatment for the edema or the ROM problem, so why mention these measurements? What do they have to do with the crutch walking? Does not talk about where pt. is independent crutch walker: in hospital? in community? in home? What is the LTG?

Plan: Is a PT involved? When will pt. be discharged? How many more treatment sessions? This note does not describe a quality or thorough treatment session.

4. **Progress Note 1:**

This is a poor note. It does not follow any of the guidelines for quality documentation. It talks about what the therapist did, in vague terms, and does not relate to the problems or how the patient is progressing. Information is organized properly and legal guidelines have been followed.

Progress Note 2:

Large space at end of S section that needs a line drawn through. Better description of treatment, but treatment cannot be duplicated accurately. Target tissue for US not identified, position of patient, type of application (direct contact or immersion). Discussion of stretching exercises does not indicate patient's position or repetitions. We do not know whether the ROM was active or passive. We do not know how far pt. ambulated, quality of gait and posture, type of surfaces. We really don't know whether US and exercise increased ankle ROM. Maybe only the US helped, or maybe only the exercise helped. Goal of independent ambulation doesn't tell reader where or how far the ambulation is required. Cannot measure this goal. Plan does not state frequency or duration or thoughts as to what will happen next session to progress the pt. It is good to see a PT involved.

Progress Note 3:

US treatment description much better. Position of pt. not mentioned, but reader could assume that the pt. was sitting because it was immersion US. Pain rating belongs in the subjective section. Stretching exercises still cannot be duplicated because we do not know patient's position or number of repetitions pt. tolerated. Nice visual for comparison of ROM measurements. We do not know what position was used when measurements were taken. We still do not know if it is AROM or PROM. A better description of the exercise program and purpose. Can visualize the patient ambulating and understand the relationship between the ankle problem and the gait. Which is more effective, US or exercise or both? What is planned for next session? How many more sessions will the pt. receive?

Progress Note 4:

Excellent note. Needs some punctuation in the first sentence. Reader can duplicate US treatment and even know which machine to use (1 MHz). Demonstration of US effectiveness. We still do not know patient's positioning for stretching exercises, but can now assume patient was sitting. We continue not to know whether ROM measurements were taken with patient sitting or in another position and whether it was active or passive ROM. An insurance representative can see that the treatment is effective in progressing the patient toward independent functioning and taking responsibility for his or her own exercises. The reader is also told that the treatments will not go on for long, but an anticipated discharge date is soon.

5. Legal guidelines followed. Subjective data appropriate. Able to reproduce stretching exercises and knee measurements. Measurements compared with previous ones. Able to visualize the patient ambulating. Observed the independent use of walker in the patient's environment to confirm the subjective information. Treatment relates to the problems; transfers/ambulation and knee stretching were described. Assessment section relates relevance of increased knee flexion to function and measures progress toward goals. Plan does not tell reader frequency or duration of remaining treatment sessions.

6. (Note from Chapter 4 Practice Exercise 3)

11-17-92 **Dx:** L CVA.

Pr: R hemiparesis interfering with safe transfers, ambulation, and independent ADLs.

Pt. admits she has not been doing her home exercise program. Does not feel like going out to church or her club meetings because she is afraid of falling. Pt. practiced transferring from floor to chair 3× with minimum assistance to help push up from kneeling position to chair seat to enable her to get up if she were to fall. Pt. required frequent verbal cuing for sequencing the movements required to roll and sit up; demonstrated inability to bear wt. on R hand due to mild flexion contractures in all finger joints, and was able to independently move from supine to sit by rolling to R side, use R elbow for support, and push up to sitting with LUE. ~~PROM~~ ^{11-17-92 ml} AAROM exercises/supine on floor/for all RUE motions/10 reps each/requiring minimal physical assistance but many verbal cues. Pt. demonstrated isometric shoulder exercises sitting, but required many reminders not to lean trunk. Pt. has difficulty remembering transfer and exercise instructions. Making slow progress toward goal of safe transfers. Treatment to continue 3×/week for 1 week and will schedule interim evaluation with PT for 11-24-92.

—Marianne Lukan, PTA

7. 1. **7-17-95 Pr:** Decreased ROM & strength RLE limiting ambulation, Ⓘ transfers and bed mobility.

Pt. stated he was able to sit on a high stool in the tub, swing his leg over and then stand to take a shower today with wife standing by to help swing his leg. He denied pain today, but reported experiencing intense muscle spasms after sitting in his easy chair, also feeling a "clink" in hip area with his extension exercise. Pt. ambulated through all rooms on first floor with one crutch on L, demonstrating good balance, erect posture, 3 point step-through gait, with supervision for verbal cues for heel–toe gait. Ⓘ stairs in home and porch, using one crutch and railing. Correctly performed 10 reps each ROM and strengthening exercises: standing at kitchen counter—toe raises, partial knee bends, hip abd., gentle hyperextension, hamstring curls; supine—SLR with approx 60–70% assist, bent knee abd.; sitting—long arc quads. Recommended he stop the hyperextension exercise if he feels "clink" again. Suggested they have easy chair raised by putting on platform and use 2 crutches when fatigued. Pt. smiling and pleasant, no longer presents with flat affect. Goal #3 met, but exercises ready to be progressed and pt. needs powder board for hip abduction. Progressing quickly toward goals 1 and 2, may be able to go to a cane, continues to need assist lifting R leg when transferring. Will bring powder board next visit on 7-25-95, monitor exercise program, and continue toward goals in PT's initial eval.

—Joe Jones, PTA

7. 2. Draw lines through long spaces at end of sentences.

Good that subjective statement is in quotation marks.
Pain complaint should go in subjective section. Better to have pt. rate the pain on a scale.
Note is about what the PTA did, not how the pt. performed. Cannot picture the patient and cannot duplicate the treatment. Need to describe how pt. looks when ambulating, how much assistance needed and why, how far or for how long ambulating, type of surfaces, assistance required on stairs. Need to describe the exercises or refer to copy in chart. Statement about pt. telling PTA how much wt. he is bearing belongs in subjective section. (PTA should measure or determine how much pt. is wt. bearing.)
No evidence in the S or O sections to support the A comments. How did PTA determine the progress was 90%? Why does pt. need 2 more visits?

7. 3. This note follows all the guidelines.
7. 4. a. Impairments: decreased strength, ROM, endurance.
     Functional limitations: transfers, bed mobility, sit ↔ stand, ambulation.
  b. (1) Safe and Ⓘ transfers from variety of surfaces in home in 3 weeks.
     (2) Safe and Ⓘ household ambulation with appropriate ambulation device for 5 or more minutes, up/down stairs to exit home in 3 weeks.
     (3) Wife/pt. to carry out home exercise program correctly and Ⓘ in 1 week.
  c. (1) Home program of ROM and strengthening exercises to increase ROM and strength of RLE to allow safe and Ⓘ transfers.
     (2) Structured home ambulation program to increase ambulation endurance to 5 min and to improve safety.
     (3) Gait training on stairs to allow exist from home.
     (4) Transfer training from a variety of surfaces with emphasis on getting in/out of bed.

Treatment will be 2×/week for 3 weeks.
Impairments will be treated by exercises to increase strength & ROM and structured, progressive ambulation to increase endurance.
Functional activities are transfers from variety of surfaces, ambulation, and stair climbing.

8. 1. There are subjective data reported from nursing only. There are no subjective data from the patient. Because pt. was confused, the subjective data would not be relevant.
8. 2. Yes, the objective data paint a picture of the wounds by describing how they look and giving measurements.
8. 3. Yes, the data are reproducible. Another PT could describe the same appearances and perform the same measurements, although measurement on R does not describe the boundaries of the measurements.
8. 4. Impairments are the pressure ulcers/open wounds with necrotic tissue and blister.
8. 5. Functional limitations are dependent bed mobility and transfers.

8. 6. Purpose of the treatment is to clean the wound of necrotic tissue and loose skin, enhance healing. Pt. should be able to improve in bed mobility and to perform assisted standing transfers when heels are healed.

8. 7. Frequency = 1×/day, and duration = 3 days.

8. 8. Debride necrotic tissue ~~in 3 days~~ for <u>clean wound with healthy tissue</u> to enhance healing for eventual assisted bed mobility and assisted pivot transfers.

8. 9. Yes, I can duplicate the treatment if I follow standard Pulsavac procedure. I know to do the treatment at bedside, and where to position towels. I also know sterile technique was used, since I am told the towels were sterile.

   There are only 3 treatments planned, so I will have the PT do the discharge eval. on the third treatment.

   I can document progress by describing how the wounds look and compare that description with the initial eval. I can measure and compare the measurements, and I can put the descriptions and measurements in chart form with initial eval. data listed for comparison.

9. 1. Documentation is evidence that may be needed years later.

9. 2. Documentation is a legal record.

9. 3. Medicare influenced history of documentation.

9. 4. Legal guidelines.

9. 5. Topic of impairment, functional limitation, and disability introduced.

9. 6. Poor documentation raises questions and makes it difficult to recall information

9. 7. How good documentation should look. A peek at what the book is about and how the student will be expected to document.

9. 8. Abbreviations.

9. 9. SOAP format.

9. 10. Recording of license number.

9. 11. Introduction to history of documentation.

9. 12. Standards and criteria mentioned.

Guidelines for Physical Therapy Documentation*

INTRODUCTION

The American Physical Therapy Association (APTA) is committed to meeting the physical therapy needs of society, to meeting the needs and interests of its members, and to developing and improving the art and science of physical therapy, including practice, education, and research. To help meet these responsibilities, the APTA Board of Directors has approved the following guidelines for physical therapy documentation. It is recognized that these guidelines do not reflect all of the unique documentation requirements associated with the many specialty areas within the physical therapy profession. These guidelines are intended to be used as a foundation for the development of more specific documentation guidelines in specialty areas, while at the same time providing guidance for the physical therapy profession across all practice settings.

OPERATIONAL DEFINITIONS

GUIDELINES APTA defines "guidelines" as approved, nonbinding statements of advice.

DOCUMENTATION Any entry into the client record, such as: consultation report, initial examination report, progress note, flowsheet/checklist that identifies the care/service provided, reexamination report, or summation of care.

I. General Guidelines
A. All documentation must comply with the applicable jurisdictional/regulatory requirements.
 1. All handwritten entries should be made in ink.
 2. Informed consent shall be obtained as required by the APTA Standards of Practice.
  2.1 The physical therapist has sole responsibility for providing information to the patient and for obtaining the patient's informed consent in accordance with jurisdictional law before initiating physical therapy.

---

*These guidelines were developed by a subgroup of APTA's Advisory Panel on Documentation and were adopted by APTA's Board of Directors in 1993.

APTA thanks Karl Gibson, MS, PT; Stephen Haley, PhD, PT; and Robert Babbs, MPA, PT, for their work in researching and preparing these guidelines.

Guidelines for Physical Therapy Documentation BOD 03-905-23-61 [Amended BOD 11-94-33-107; BOD 06-93-09-13; Adopted BOD 03-93-21-55]

From American Physical Therapy Association: American Physical Therapy Association Guidelines: Guidelines for Physical Therapy Documentation. APTA, Alexandria, VA, 1995, pp 1–10, with permission of the APTA.

2.2 Those deemed competent to give consent are competent adults. When the adult is not competent, and in the case of minors, a parent or legal guardian consents as the surrogate decision maker.

2.3 The information provided to the patient should include the following: (a) a clear description of the treatment ordered or recommended, (b) material (decisional) risks associated with the proposed treatment, (c) expected benefits of treatment, (d) comparison of the benefits and risks possible with and without treatment, and (e) reasonable alternatives to the recommended treatment. The physical therapist should solicit questions from the patient and provide answers. The patient should be asked to acknowledge understanding and consent before treatment proceeds.

Examples of ways in which to accomplish this documentation:

2.3.1 Signature of patient/guardian on long or short consent form,

2.3.2 Notation/entry of what was explained by the physical therapist or the physical therapist assistant in the official record, and

2.3.3 Filing of a completed consent checklist signed by the patient.

3. Charting errors should be corrected by drawing a single line through the error and initialing and dating the chart.

4. Identification

4.1 Include patient's full name and identification number, if applicable, on all official documents.

4.2 All entries must be dated and signed with the provider's full name and appropriate designation (eg, PT, PTA).

4.3 Documentation by students (SPT/SPTA) shall be countersigned by a licensed physical therapist.

4.4 Documentation by graduates (GPT/GPTA) or others pending receipt of an unrestricted license shall be countersigned by a licensed physical therapist.

5. Documentation should include the manner in which physical therapy services are initiated.

Examples include

5.1 Self-referral/direct access,

5.2 Attachment of the referral/consultation request by a qualified practitioner, and

5.3 File copy of correspondence to referral source as acknowledgement of the referral.

II. Initial Examination and Evaluation/Consultation

A. Documentation is required at the onset of each episode of physical therapy care.

B. Elements include:

1. Obtaining a history and identifying risk factors

1.1 History of the presenting problem, current complaints, and precautions (including onset date).

1.2 Pertinent diagnoses and medical history.

1.3 Demographic characteristics, including pertinent psychological, social, and environmental factors.

1.4 Prior or concurrent services related to the current episode of physical therapy care.

1.5 Comorbidities that may affect goals and treatment plan.

1.6 Statement of patient's knowledge of problem.

1.7 Goals of patient (and family members and significant others, if appropriate).

2. Selecting and administering tests and measures to determine patient status in a number of areas. The following is a partial list of these areas, with illustrative tests and measures:

2.1 Arousal, mentation, and cognition.

Examples include objective findings related, but not limited, to the following areas:

2.1.1 Level of consciousness,

2.1.2 Ability to process commands,

2.1.3 Alertness, and

2.1.4 Gross expressive and receptive deficits.

2.2 Neuromotor development and sensory integration.

Examples include objective findings related, but not limited, to the following areas:

2.2.1 Gross and fine motor skills,

2.2.2 Reflex and movement patterns, and

2.2.3 Dexterity, agility, and coordination.

2.3 Range of motion.

Examples include objective findings related, but not limited, to the following areas:

2.3.1 Extent of joint motion,

2.3.1 Pain and soreness of surrounding soft tissue, and

2.3.2 Muscle length and flexibility.

2.4 Muscle performance.

Examples include objective findings related, but not limited, to the following areas:

2.4.1 Strength,

2.4.2 Power, and

2.4.3 Endurance.

2.5 Ventilation, respiration, and circulation.

Examples include objective findings related, but not limited, to the following areas:

2.5.1 Vital signs,

2.5.2 Breathing patterns, and

2.5.3 Heart sounds.

2.6 Posture.

Examples include objective findings related, but not limited, to the following areas:

2.6.1 Static posture, and

2.6.2 Dynamic posture.

2.7 Gait and balance.

Examples include objective findings related, but not limited, to the following areas:

2.7.1 Characteristics of gait,

2.7.2 Functional ambulation, and

2.7.3 Characteristics of balance.

2.8 Self-care or home-management status.

Examples include objective findings related, but not limited, to the following areas:

2.8.1 Activities of daily living,

2.8.2 Functional capacity, and

2.8.3 Static and dynamic strength.

2.9 Community or work reintegration.

Examples include objective findings related, but not limited, to the following areas:

2.9.1 Instrumental activities of daily living,

2.9.3 Functional capacity, and

2.9.3 Adaptive skills.

2.10 Other characteristics of patient performance (eg, integumentary integrity, aerobic capacity, or endurance).

3. Evaluation (a dynamic process in which the physical therapist makes clinical judgments based on data gathered during the examination).

4. Diagnosis (a label encompassing a cluster of signs and symptoms, syndromes, or categories that reflects the information obtained from the examination).

5. Goals

5.1 Patient (and family members and significant others, if appropriate) is involved in establishing goals.

5.2 All goals are stated in measurable terms.

5.3 Goals are linked to problems identified in the examination.

5.4 Short- and long-term goals are established when applicable. (May include potential for achieving goals.)

6. Intervention plan or recommendation requirements

6.1 Shall be related to realistic goals and expected functional outcomes.

6.2 Should include frequency (eg, two times per week) and duration (eg, 3 weeks) to achieve the stated goals.

6.3 Should include patient and family/caregiver educational goals.

6.4 Should involve appropriate collaboration and coordination of care with other professionals/services.

7. Signature and appropriate designation of physical therapist.

III. Documentation of the Continuum of Care

A. Intervention or service provided.

1. Documentation is required for each patient visit/encounter. Examples include:

1.1 Checklist,

1.2 Flow sheet,

1.3 Graph, and

1.4 Narrative.

2. Elements include:

2.1 Identification of specific interventions provided,

2.2 Equipment provided, and

2.3 Signature and appropriate designation, or initials, of:

2.3.1 The physical therapist, physical therapist assistant, or other personnel providing the service under the supervision of a physical therapist; or

2.3.2 The physical therapist who supervised the provision of service

B. Patient status, progress, or regression

1. Documentation is required weekly for patients seen at intervals of 1 week or less. If the patient is seen less frequently, documentation is required for every visit/encounter.

2. Elements include:

2.1 Subjective status of patient.

2.2 Changes in objective and measurable findings as they relate to existing goals.

2.3 Adverse reaction to treatment.

2.4 Progression/regression of existing therapeutic regimen, including patient education and compliance.

2.5 Communication/consultation with providers/patient/family/significant other.

2.6 Signature and appropriate designation of either a physical therapist or a physical therapist assistant.

C. Reexamination and reevaluation.

1. Documentation is required monthly for patients seen at intervals of 1 month or less. If the patient is seen less frequently, documentation is required for every visit/encounter.

2. Elements include:

2.1 Documentation of elements as identified in III.B.2.1 through III.B.2.5 to update patient's status.

      2.2 Interpretation of findings and, when indicated, revision of goals.

      2.3 When indicated, revision of treatment plan, as directly correlated with documented goals.

      2.4 Signature and appropriate designation of physical therapist.

IV. Summation of Care

  A. Documentation is required following conclusion of the current episode in the physical therapy care sequence.

  B. Elements include:

    1. Reason for discontinuation of service.

    Examples include:

      1.1 Satisfactory goal achievement.

      1.2 Patient declines to continue care.

      1.3 Patient is unable to continue to work toward goals because of medical or psychosocial complications.

      1.4 Physical therapist determines that the patient will no longer benefit from physical therapy services.

    2. Current physical/functional status.

    3. Degree of goal achievement and reasons for goals not being achieved.

    4. Discharge plan that includes written and verbal communication related to the patient's continuing care.

    Examples include:

      4.1 Home program,

      4.2 Referrals for additional services,

      4.3 Recommendations for follow-up physical therapy care,

      4.4 Family and caregiver training, and

      4.5 Equipment provided.

    5. Signature and appropriate designation of physical therapist.

Index

Page numbers followed by an "f" indicate a figure; page numbers followed by a "t" indicate a table.